Super-Easy Anti-Inflammatory Dishes for Busy People

Anti-Inflammatory Recipes to Create your Tasty and Healthy Meals

Thomas Jollif

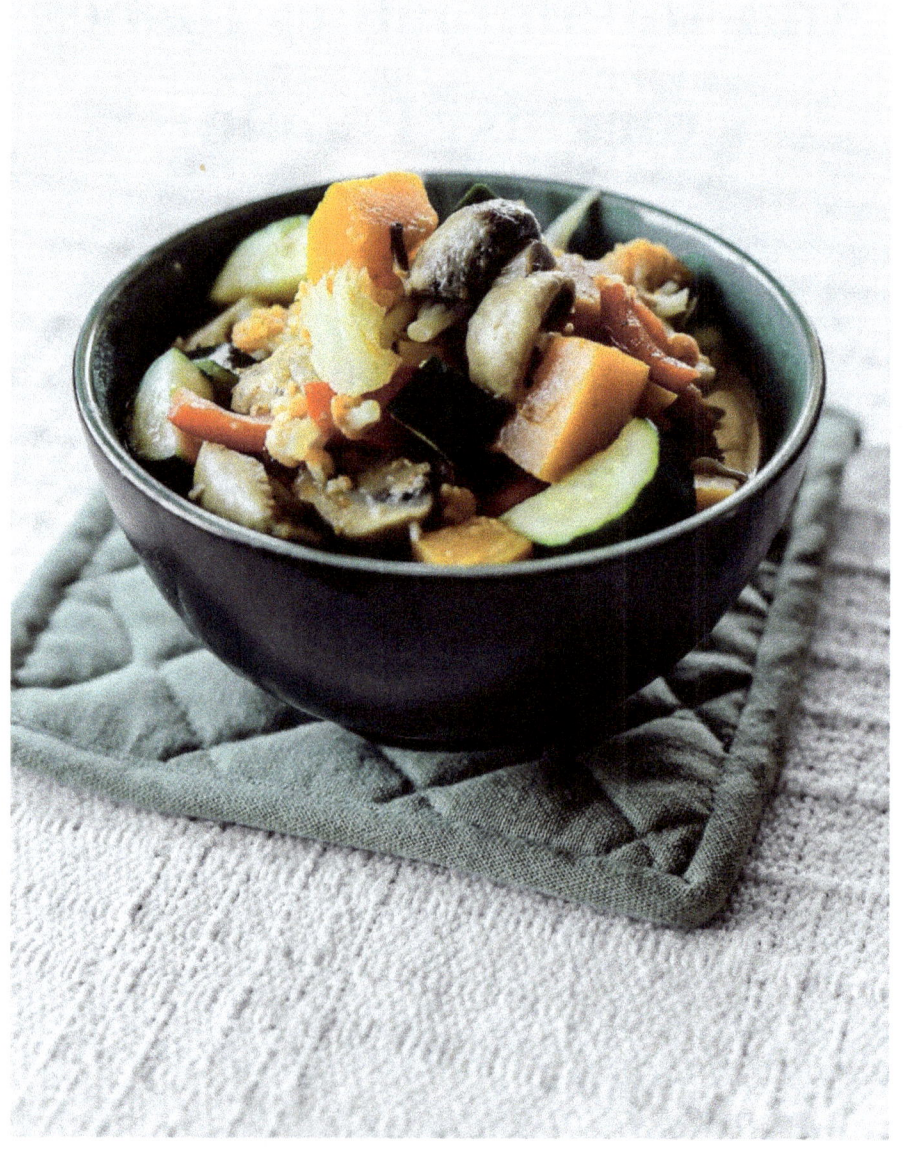

© copyright 2021 – all rights reserved.

the content contained within this book may not be reproduced, duplicated or transmitted without direct written permission from the author or the publisher.

under no circumstances will any blame or legal responsibility be held against the publisher, or author, for any damages, reparation, or monetary loss due to the information contained within this book. either directly or indirectly.

legal notice:

this book is copyright protected. this book is only for personal use. you cannot amend, distribute, sell, use, quote or paraphrase any part, or the content within this book, without the consent of the author or publisher.

disclaimer notice:

please note the information contained within this document is for educational and entertainment purposes only. all effort has been executed to present accurate, up to date, and reliable, complete information. no warranties of any kind are declared or implied. readers acknowledge that the author is not engaging in the rendering of legal, financial, medical or professional advice. the content within this book has been derived from various sources. please consult a licensed professional before attempting any techniques outlined in this book.

by reading this document, the reader agrees that under no circumstances is the author responsible for any losses, direct or indirect, which are incurred as a result of the use of information contained within this document, including, but not limited to, — errors, omissions, or inaccuracies.

Table of Contents

BREAKFASTS 7
- CINNAMON-APPLE GRANOLA WITH GREEK YOGURT 7
- COCONUT & BANANA COOKIES 9
- COCO-TAPIOCA BOWL 11
- CORNMEAL GRITS 12
- CRANBERRY AND RAISINS GRANOLA 14
- CREAM CHEESE SALMON TOAST 16
- CREPES WITH COCONUT CREAM & STRAWBERRY SAUCE 18
- EDAMAME OMELET 21
- EGG MUFFINS WITH FETA AND QUINOA 23
- FANTASTIC SPAGHETTI SQUASH WITH CHEESE AND BASIL PESTO 25

SMOOTHIES AND DRINKS 27
- DREAMY YUMMY ORANGE CREAM SMOOTHIE 27
- FIG SMOOTHIE 29
- FLU FIGHTING TONIC 31
- FRESH CRANBERRY AND LIME JUICE 32
- FRESH TROPICAL JUICE 34
- GINGER ALE 36
- GINGER, CARROT, AND TURMERIC SMOOTHIE 38
- GOLDEN CHAI LATTE 40

SIDES 42
- GOAT CHEESE SALAD 42
- GREEN BEANS 45
- GREEN, RED AND YELLOW RICE 47

HOT PINK COCONUT SLAW 49

SAUCES AND DRESSINGS 51

CREAMY RASPBERRY VINAIGRETTE 51
CREAMY SIAMESE DRESSING 53

SNACKS 55

CASHEW CHEESE 55
CAULIFLOWER SNACKS 57
CEREAL CHIA CHIPS 59
CHEWY BLACKBERRY LEATHER 61
CHIA CASHEW CREAM 63
COCO CHERRY BAKE-LESS BARS 64
COCONUT PORRIDGE 66

SOUPS AND STEWS 68

CREAMY LEEK SOUP 68
CREAMY PARSNIP SOUP 70
CREAMY PUMPKIN PUREE SOUP 72
CREAMY TURKEY SOUP 74
CREAMY TURMERIC CAULIFLOWER SOUP 75
CROCK-POT TURKEY TACO SOUP 77
DETOX CABBAGE SOUP 79
FENNEL AND PEAR SOUP 81
FRENCH CARAMELIZED ONION SOUP 83
GARLIC AND LENTIL SOUP 85

DESSERTS 87

CHOCOLATE MOUSSE 87
CINNAMON APPLE CHIPS 89

CITRUS CAULIFLOWER CAKE 91
CITRUS STRAWBERRY GRANITA 94
COCONUT AND CHOCOLATE CREAM 96
COCONUT BUTTER FUDGE 98
COCONUT MUFFINS... 99
COFFEE CREAM 101
COMFORTING BAKED RICE PUDDING 103
COOKIE DOUGH BITES.. 105

BREAKFASTS

Cinnamon-Apple Granola with Greek Yogurt

Time To Prepare: five minutes
Time to Cook: ten minutes
Yield: Servings 2

Ingredients:

- ½ apple, peeled and diced
- ½ c. raw almonds, chopped (or raw nuts of choice)
- ½ c. raw walnuts, chopped (or raw nuts of choice)
- 1 cup Greek plain or vanilla yogurt (or flavor of choice)
- 1 tbsp. almond flour
- 1 tsp. ground cinnamon
- 1/16 tsp. vanilla extract
- 1/8 c. applesauce, unsweetened preferred
- 2 tbsp. vanilla Protein powder
- 2 tsp. almond butter
- 2 tsp. honey
- dash of sea salt

Directions:

1. In a mixing container, mix the chopped almonds, chopped walnuts (or preferred raw nuts), diced apple, vanilla Protein powder, almond flour, lucuma (opt), and cinnamon and salt in a container. Mix thoroughly.
2. In a second container, mix the apple sauce, almond butter, honey, and vanilla extract. Mix thoroughly. Pour the container with the nuts into the container with the wet ingredients and blend together meticulously. Make sure all dry ingredients get coated.
3. Put the granola mixture onto a parchment paperlined baking sheet and bake until the desired crunch is obtained roughly 8 to ten minutes. Take off from oven and allow to cool or eat hot. Put ½ cup each Greek yogurt into two bowls. Split the granola and drizzle over the yogurt in each container. Serve instantly.

Nutritional Info: Calories: 312 kcal ‖ Protein: 11.72 g ‖ Fat: 22.37 g ‖ Carbohydrates: 19.92 g

Coconut & Banana Cookies

Time To Prepare: fifteen minutes
Time to Cook: twenty-five minutes
Yield: Servings 7

Ingredients:

- ½ tsp. ground cinnamon
- ½ tsp. ground turmeric
- 2 cups unsweetened coconut, shredded
- 3 medium bananas, peeled
- Freshly ground black pepper
- Pinch of salt, to taste

Directions:

1. Set the oven to 350°F. Coat a cookie sheet a mildly greased parchment paper.
2. In a mixer, put all together ingredients and pulse till a dough-like mixture forms.
3. Make small balls through the mixture and set onto a prepared cookie sheet in a single layer.
4. Using your fingers, press along the balls to form the cookies.
5. Bake for minimum fifteen-twenty minutes or till golden brown.

Nutritional Info: Calories: 370 ‖ Fat: 4g ‖ Carbohydrates: 28g ‖ Fiber: 11g ‖ Protein: 33g

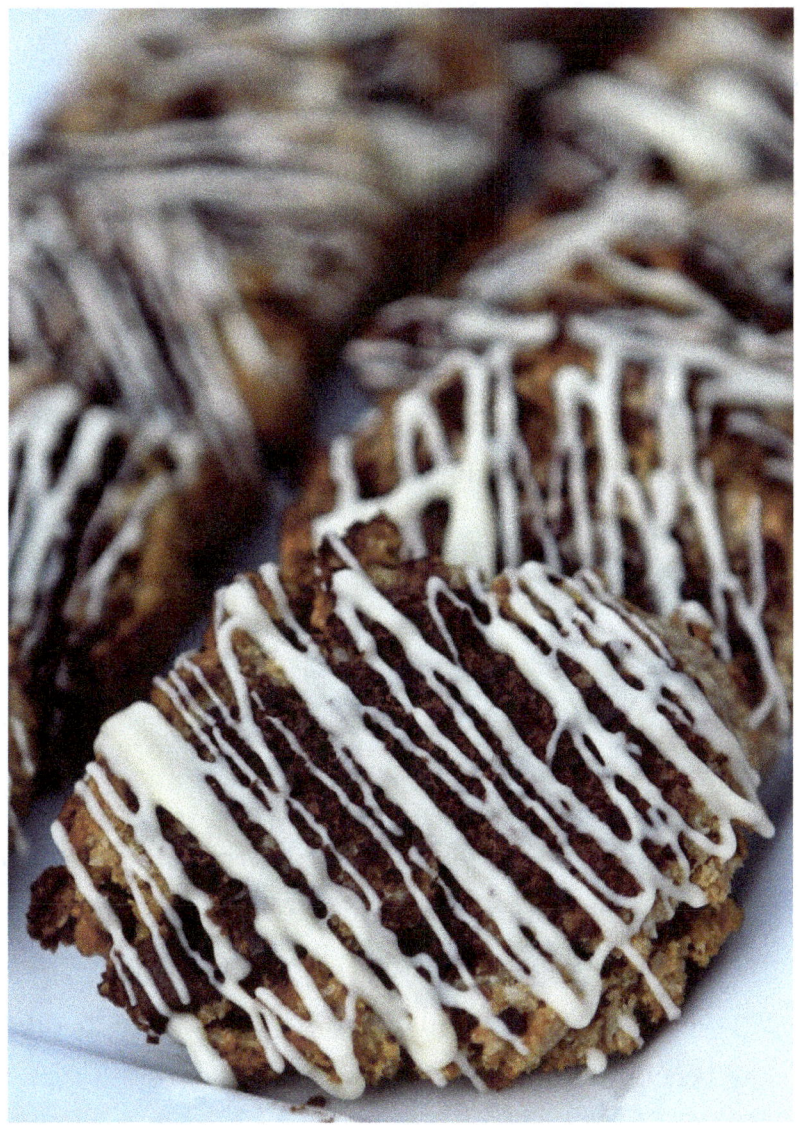

Coco-Tapioca Bowl

Time To Prepare: ten minutes
Time to Cook: twenty minutes
Yield: Servings 2
Ingredients:

- ¼ cup maple syrup
- ¼ cup tapioca pearls, small sized
- ½ cup unsweetened coconut flakes, toasted
- 1 ½ tsp. lemon juice
- 1 can light coconut milk
- 2 cups water

Directions:

1. Put the tapioca in a deep cooking pan and pour over the 2 cups of water. Allow it to stand for minimum 30 minutes.
2. Pour in the coconut milk and syrup and heat the deep cooking pan over moderate temperature. Bring to its boiling point while stirring continuously.
3. Put in the lemon juice and stir and then decorate with coconut flakes.

Nutritional Info: Calories: 309 kcal ‖ Protein: 3.93 g ‖ Fat: 9.02 g ‖ Carbohydrates: 54.55 g

Cornmeal Grits

Time To Prepare: five minutes
Time to Cook: fifteen minutes
Yield: Servings 4

Ingredients:

- 1 cup polenta meal
- 1 teaspoon salt
- 2 tablespoons butter
- 4 cups water

Directions:

1. Put water and salt in a deep cooking pan then place it to its boiling point.
2. Slowly put in polenta and continuously stir on moderate to low heat until it has become thick, approximately fifteen minutes. Mix in butter.
3. Serve instantly for tender grits or pour into a greased loaf pan and allow to cool.
4. Once cool, grits can be cut and fried or grilled.

Nutritional Info: Calories: 177 ‖ Fat: 6 g ‖ Protein: 3 g ‖ Sodium: 641 mg ‖ Fiber: 2.5 g ‖ Carbohydrates: 27 g

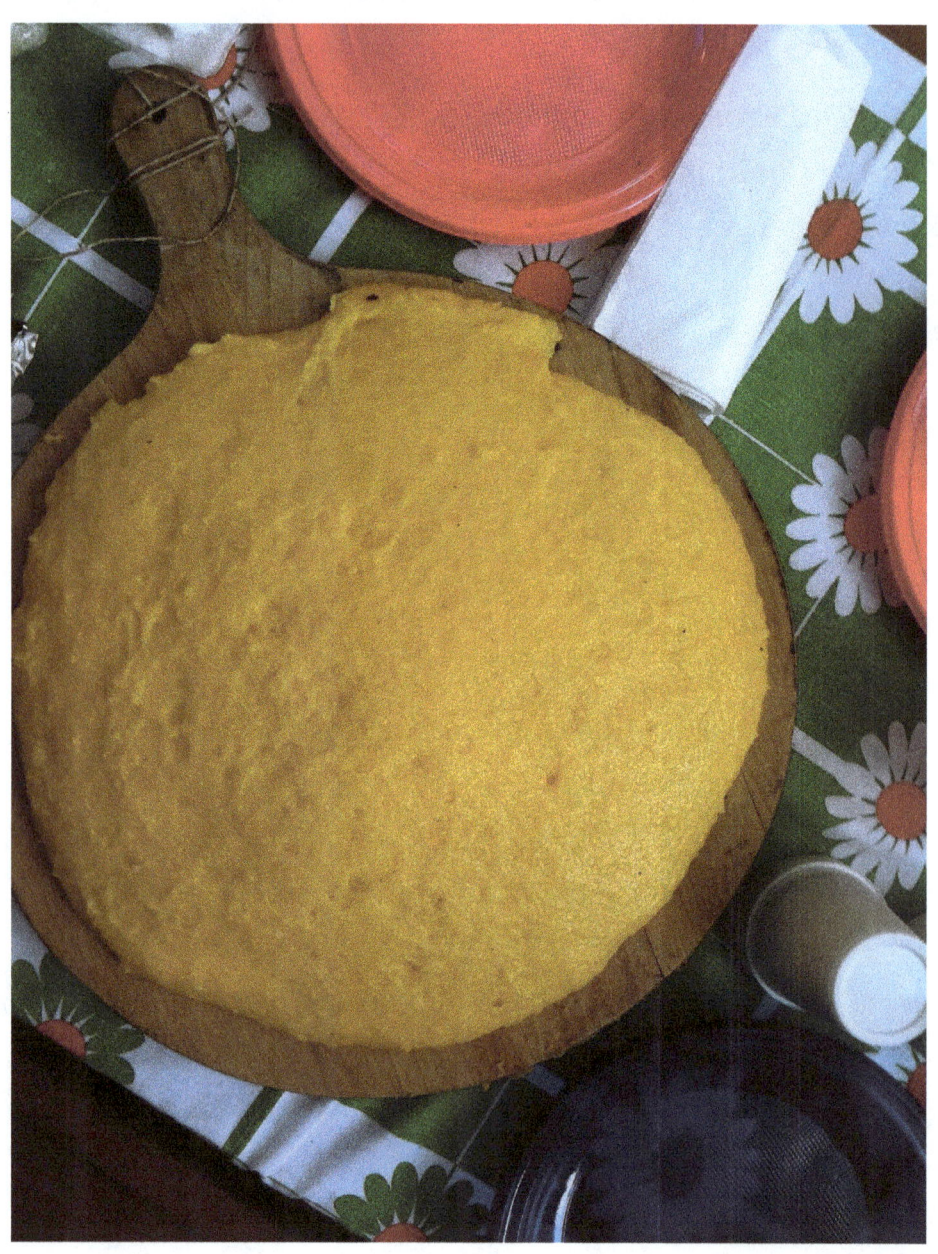

Cranberry and Raisins Granola

Time To Prepare: fifteen minutes
Time to Cook: twenty minutes
Yield: Servings 4

Ingredients:

- 4 cups old-fashioned rolled oats
- 1 cup dried cranberries
- 1 cup golden raisins
- 2 tablespoons olive oil
- ½ cup almonds, slivered
- 2 tablespoons warm water
- 1 teaspoon vanilla extract
- 1 teaspoon cinnamon
- 6 tablespoons maple syrup
- 1/3 cup of honey
- 1/4 cup sesame seeds
- 1/4 teaspoon of salt
- 1/8 teaspoon nutmeg

Directions:

1. In a container, combine the sesame seeds, nutmeg, almonds, oats, salt, and cinnamon.

2. In another container, combine the oil, water, vanilla, honey, and syrup. Slowly pour the mixture into the oats mixture. Toss to blend. Spread the mixture into a greased jelly-roll pan. Bake using your oven at 300°F for minimum 55 minutes. Stir and break the clumps every ten minutes.
3. Once you get it from the oven, stir the cranberries and raisins. Allow cooling. This will last for a week when stored in an airtight container and up to a month when stored in your refrigerator.

Nutritional Info: Calories: 698 kcal ‖ Protein: 21.34 g ‖ Fat: 20.99 g ‖ Carbohydrates: 148.59 g

Cream Cheese Salmon Toast

Time To Prepare: fifteen minutes
Time to Cook: five minutes
Yield: Servings 2

Ingredients:
- ½ cup Arugula or spinach, chopped
- ½ tsp. Basil flakes
- 1 tbsp. Red onion, chopped fine
- 2 oz. Smoked salmon
- 2 tbsp. Cream cheese, low-fat
- Whole grain or rye toast, two slices

Directions:
1. Toast the wheat bread.
2. Mix cream cheese and basil and spread this mixture on the toast.
3. Put in salmon, arugula, and onion.

Nutritional Info: Calories 291 ‖ 15.2 grams Fat (8.5 saturated) ‖ 17.8 grams Carbohydrates ‖ 3 grams of sugar

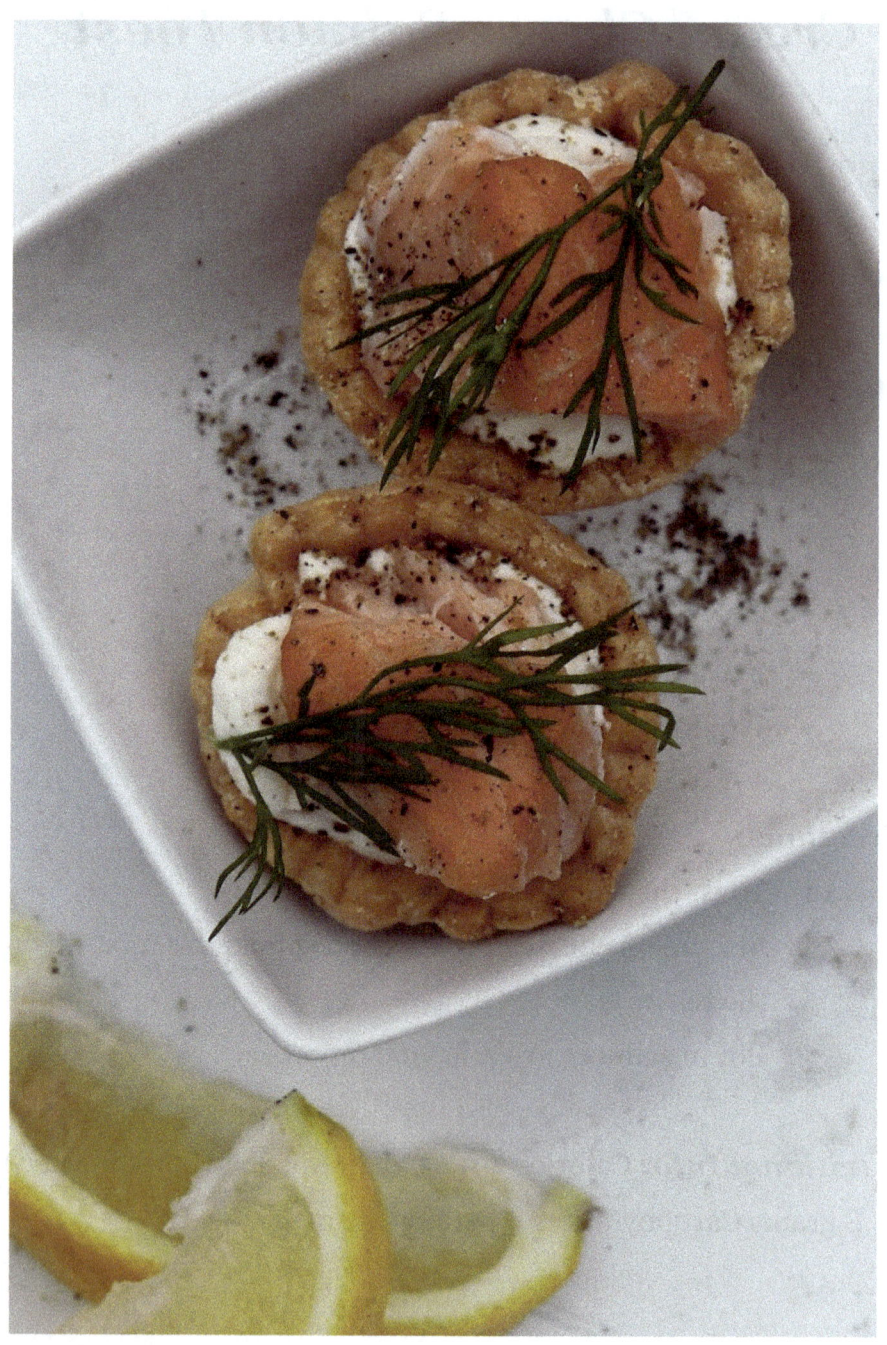

Crepes with Coconut Cream & Strawberry Sauce

Time To Prepare: fifteen minutes
Time to Cook: 8 minutes
Yield: Servings 4

Ingredients:
For Sauce:

- 1 (13½-ounce) can chilled coconut milk
- 1 tablespoon honey
- 1 tablespoon organic honey
- 1 teaspoon organic vanilla flavoring
- 1½ teaspoons tapioca starch
- 12-ounces frozen strawberries, thawed and liquid reserved
- For the Coconut cream:

For Crepes:

- ¼ cup almond milk
- 2 organic eggs
- 2 tablespoons coconut flour
- 2 tablespoons tapioca starch
- Avocado oil, as required
- Pinch of salt

Directions:

1. For sauce inside a container, combine some reserved strawberry liquid and tapioca starch.
2. Put in rest of the ingredients and mix thoroughly.
3. Move a combination inside a pan on moderate to high heat.
4. Bring to its boiling point, stirring constantly.
5. Cook for minimum 2-3 minutes, till the sauce, becomes thick.
6. Turn off the heat and aside, covered till serving.
7. For coconut cream, cautiously, scoop your cream from your surface of a can of coconut milk.
8. In a mixer, put in coconut cream, vanilla flavoring, and honey and pulse for around 6-8 minutes or till fluffy.
9. For crepes in a blender, put in all ingredients and pulse till well blended and smooth.
10. Lightly, grease a substantial nonstick frying pan with avocado oil as well as heat on medium-low heat.
11. Put in a modest amount of mixture and tilt the pan to spread it uniformly inside the frying pan.
12. Cook roughly 1-2 minutes.
13. Cautiously change the side and cook for roughly 1-1½ minutes more.
14. Repeat with the rest of the mixture.
15. Split the coconut cream onto each crepe uniformly and fold into four equivalent portions.

16. Put strawberry sauce ahead before you serve.

Nutritional Info: Calories: 364 ‖ Fat: 9g ‖ Carbohydrates: 26g ‖ Fiber: 7g ‖ Protein: 15g

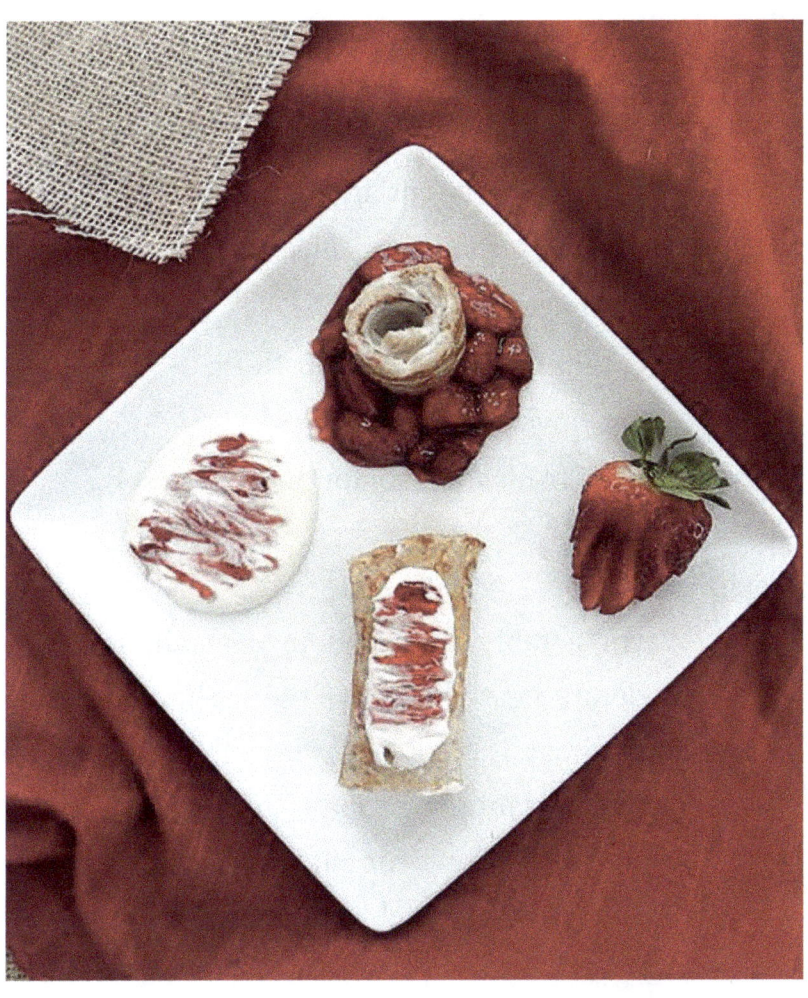

Edamame Omelet

Time To Prepare: five minutes
Time to Cook: five minutes
Yield: Servings 2

Ingredients:

- ½ cup shelled edamame
- ½ cup shredded regular or soy Cheddar cheese
- 1 bunch scallions, cut into 1-inch pieces
- 1 tbsp. low-sodium soy sauce, or to taste
- 1 tsp. minced garlic
- 3 big eggs or ¾ cup egg substitute
- 3 tbsp. olive oil, divided
- Snips of fresh cilantro, for decoration

Directions:

1. Warm 2 tablespoons oil in a small frying pan on moderate heat and sauté the garlic and scallion for approximately 2 minutes. Put in the edamame and soy sauce and sauté one minute more. Remove from the frying pan and save for later.
2. Warm the other 1 tablespoon oil in the same frying pan.

3. Whisk the eggs until combined and pour into the hot oil. Spread the shredded cheese on top. Lift up the omelet's edges, tipping the frying pan back and forth to cook the uncooked eggs.
4. Once the top looks firm, drizzle the scallion mixture over one half of the omelet and fold the other half over the top.
5. Lift the omelet out of the frying pan. Split it in half, drizzle with the cilantro, before you serve.

Nutritional Info: Calories: 416 ‖ Fat: 31 g ‖ Protein: 27 g ‖ Sodium: 640 g ‖ Fiber: 3 g ‖ Carbohydrates: 7.5 g

Egg Muffins with Feta and Quinoa

Time To Prepare: fifteen minutes
Time to Cook: thirty minutes
Yield: Servings 6-12

Ingredients:

- ¼ cup Black olives, chopped
- ¼ cup Onion, chopped
- ¼ tsp. Salt
- 1 cup Feta cheese
- 1 cup Quinoa, cooked
- 1 cup Tomatoes, chopped
- 1 tbsp. Oregano, fresh chop
- 2 cups baby spinach, chopped
- 2 tsp. Olive oil
- 8 Eggs

Directions:

1. Heat oven to 350. Spray oil a muffin pan with twelve cups. Cook spinach, oregano, olives, onion, and tomatoes for 5 minutes in the olive oil on moderate

heat. Beat eggs. Put in the cooked mix of veggies to the eggs with the cheese and salt.

2. Ladle mix into muffin cups. Bake thirty minutes. These will remain fresh in your refrigerator for two days. To eat, just wrap in a paper towel and warm in the microwave for thirty seconds.

Nutritional Info: Calorie 113 ‖ 5 grams carbs ‖ 6 grams Protein ‖ 7 grams Fat ‖ 1-gram sugar ‖

Fantastic Spaghetti Squash with Cheese and Basil Pesto

Time To Prepare: ten minutes
Time to Cook: thirty-five minutes
Yield: Servings 2

Ingredients:

- ¼ cup ricotta cheese, unsweetened
- ½ tbsp. olive oil
- 1 cup cooked spaghetti squash, drained
- 1/8 cup basil pesto
- 2oz fresh mozzarella cheese, cubed
- Freshly cracked black pepper, to taste
- Salt, to taste

Directions:

1. Switch on the oven, then set its temperature to 375 °F and allow it to preheat.
2. In the meantime, take a medium container, put in spaghetti squash in it and then sprinkle with salt and black pepper.

3. Take a casserole dish, grease it with oil, put in squash mixture in it, top it with ricotta cheese and mozzarella cheese and bake for about ten minutes until cooked.
4. When finished, remove the casserole dish from the oven, sprinkle pesto on top and serve instantly.

Nutritional Info: Calories 169 ‖ Total Fat: 11.3g ‖ Carbs: 6.2g ‖ Protein: 11.9g ‖ Sugar: 0.1g ‖ Sodium: 217mg

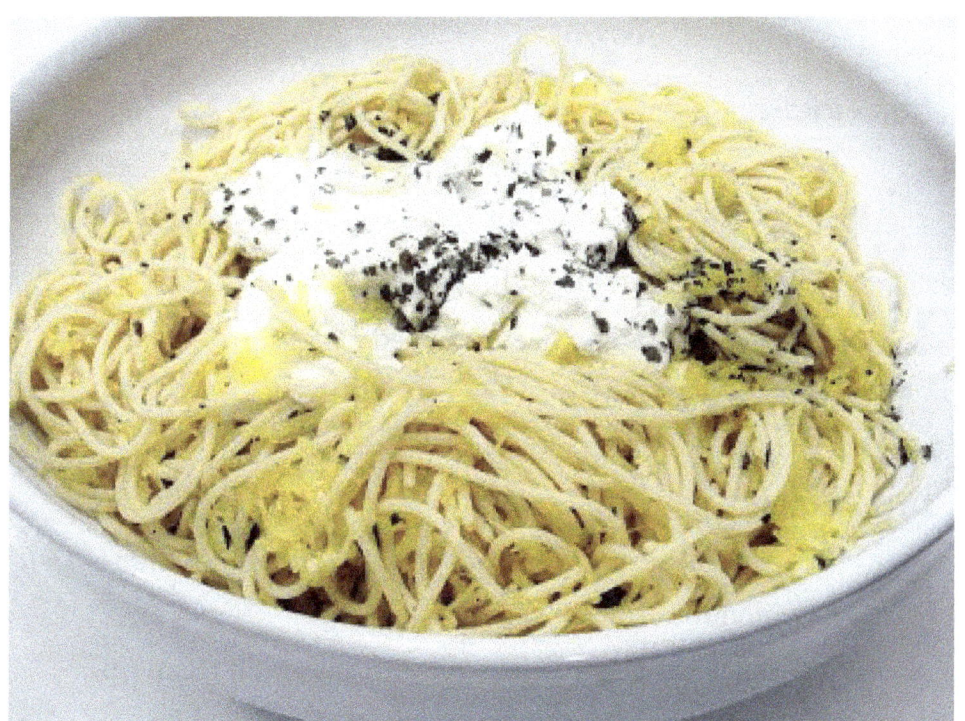

SMOOTHIES AND DRINKS

Dreamy Yummy Orange Cream Smoothie

Time To Prepare: five minutes
Time to Cook: 0 minutes
Yield: Servings 2

Ingredients:

- ¼ cup of fresh orange juice
- ½ cup of canned full-fat coconut milk
- 1 cup of almond milk
- 1 navel orange, peel removed
- 6 to 8 ice cubes

Directions:

1. Mix the smoothie ingredients in your high-speed blender.
2. Pulse the ingredients a few times to cut them up.
3. Combine the mixture on the highest speed setting for thirty to 60 seconds.
4. Pour into glasses and serve.

Nutritional Info: Calories: 269 kcal ‖ Protein: 8.63 g ‖ Fat: 21.36 g ‖ Carbohydrates: 12.75 g

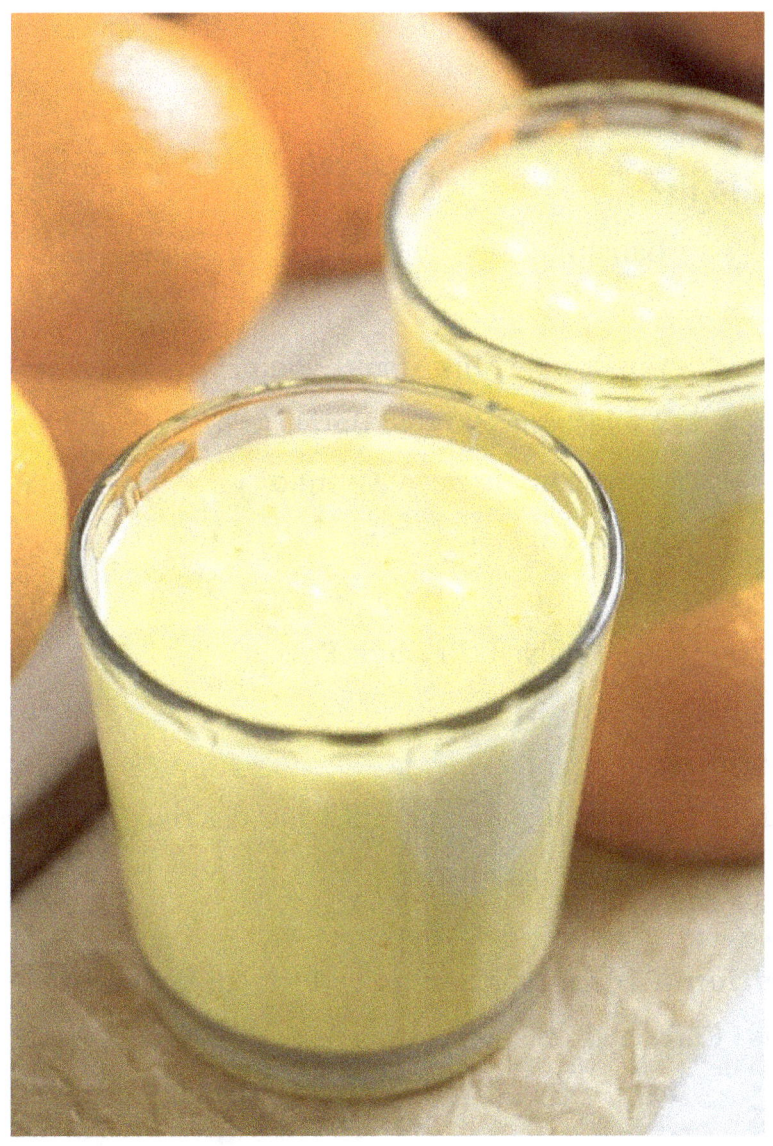

Fig Smoothie

Time To Prepare: five minutes
Time to Cook: 0 minutes
Yield: Servings 2

Ingredients:

- 1 Banana
- 1 Cup Almond Milk
- 1 Cup Whole Milk Yogurt, Plain
- 1 Tablespoon Almond Butter
- 1 Teaspoon Flaxseed, Ground
- 1 Teaspoon Honey, Raw
- 3-4 Ice Cubes
- 7 Figs, Halved (Fresh or Frozen)

Directions:

Blend all together ingredients until the desired smoothness is achieved, and serve instantly.

Nutritional Info: Calories: 362 ‖ Protein: 9 Grams ‖ Fat: 12 Grams ‖ Carbohydrates: 60 Grams

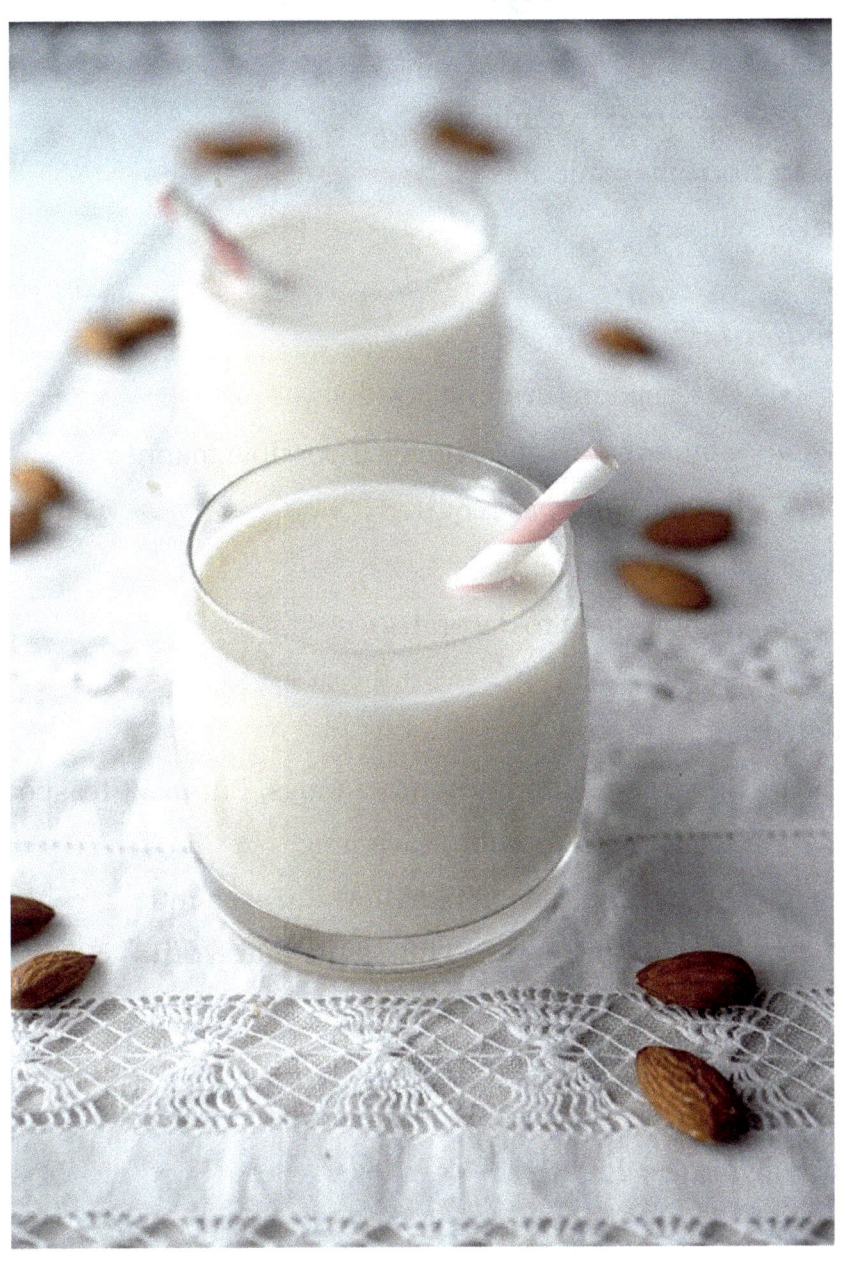

Flu Fighting Tonic

Time To Prepare: five minutes
Time to Cook: ten minutes
Yield: Servings 2

Ingredients:

- ½ teaspoon turmeric powder
- 2 tablespoons clear honey if possible manuka
- Boiling water, as required
- Juice of 2 lemons
- Lemon slices to decorate

Directions:

1. Split the lemon juice into 2 mugs. Put in ¼ teaspoon turmeric powder into each mug.
2. Put in a tablespoon of honey into each mug.
3. Pour boiling water to fill up the mugs. Stir.
4. Decorate using a slice of lemon before you serve.

Nutritional Info: Calories: 123 kcal ‖ Protein: 3.59 g ‖ Fat: 3.23 g ‖ Carbohydrates: 22.78 g

Fresh Cranberry And Lime Juice

Time To Prepare: five minutes
Time to Cook: 0 minutes
Yield: Servings 2

Ingredients:

- 1/2½ cups of mixed berries (frozen are fine)
- 1/2½ cups of spinach
- 2 limes, juiced
- 4 cups of cranberries

Directions:

Mix all the ingredients with water in a juicer until pureed and serve instantly over ice.

Nutritional Info: Calories: 578 kcal ‖ Protein: 6.83 g ‖ Fat: 9.92 g ‖ Carbohydrates: 119.35 g

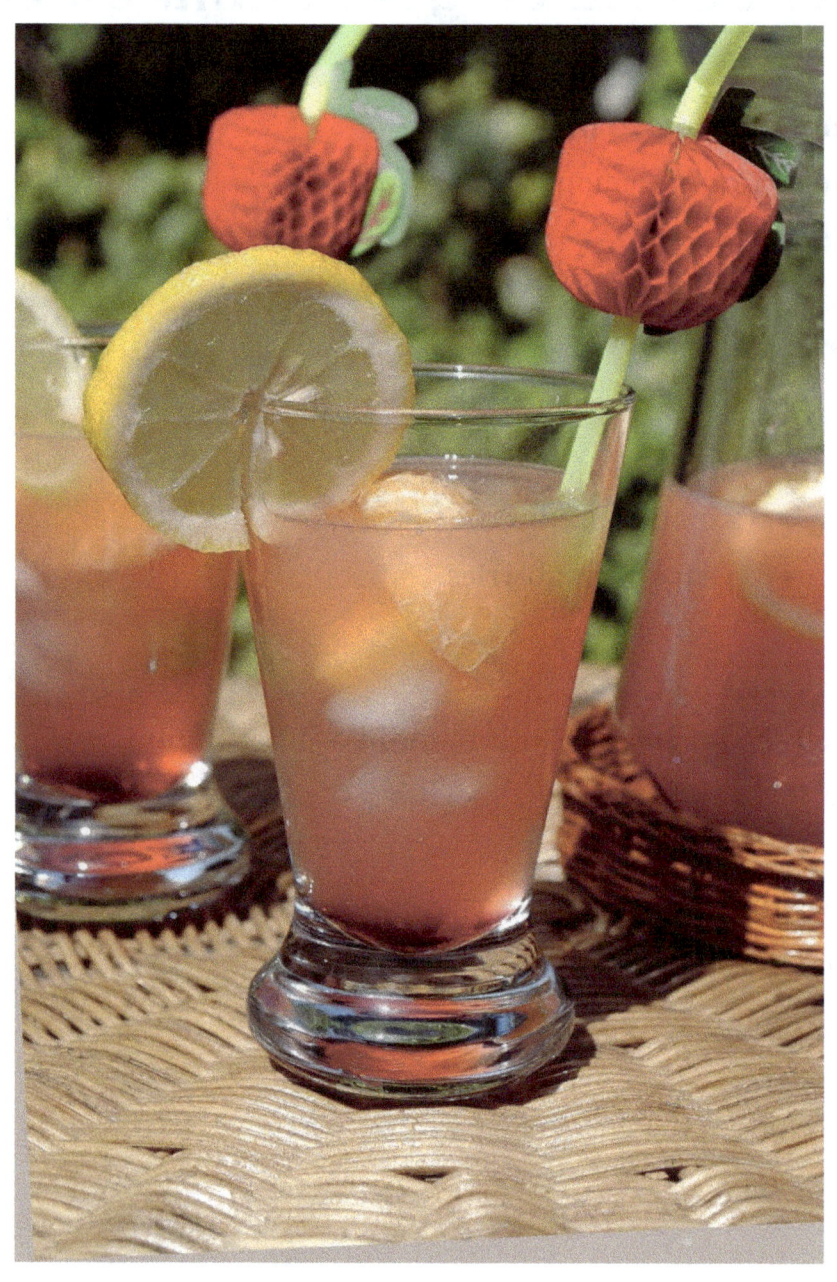

Fresh Tropical Juice

Time To Prepare: five minutes
Time to Cook: 0 minutes
Yield: Servings 2

Ingredients:

- 1 whole pineapple, peeled and slice into chunks.
- 1 cup of water
- 1/2 can of low-fat coconut milk

Directions:

1. Put in all ingredients to a juicer and blend until the desired smoothness is achieved.
2. Serve over ice.

Nutritional Info: Calories: 116 kcal ‖ Protein: 3.72 g ‖ Fat: 3.13 g ‖ Carbohydrates: 19.55 g

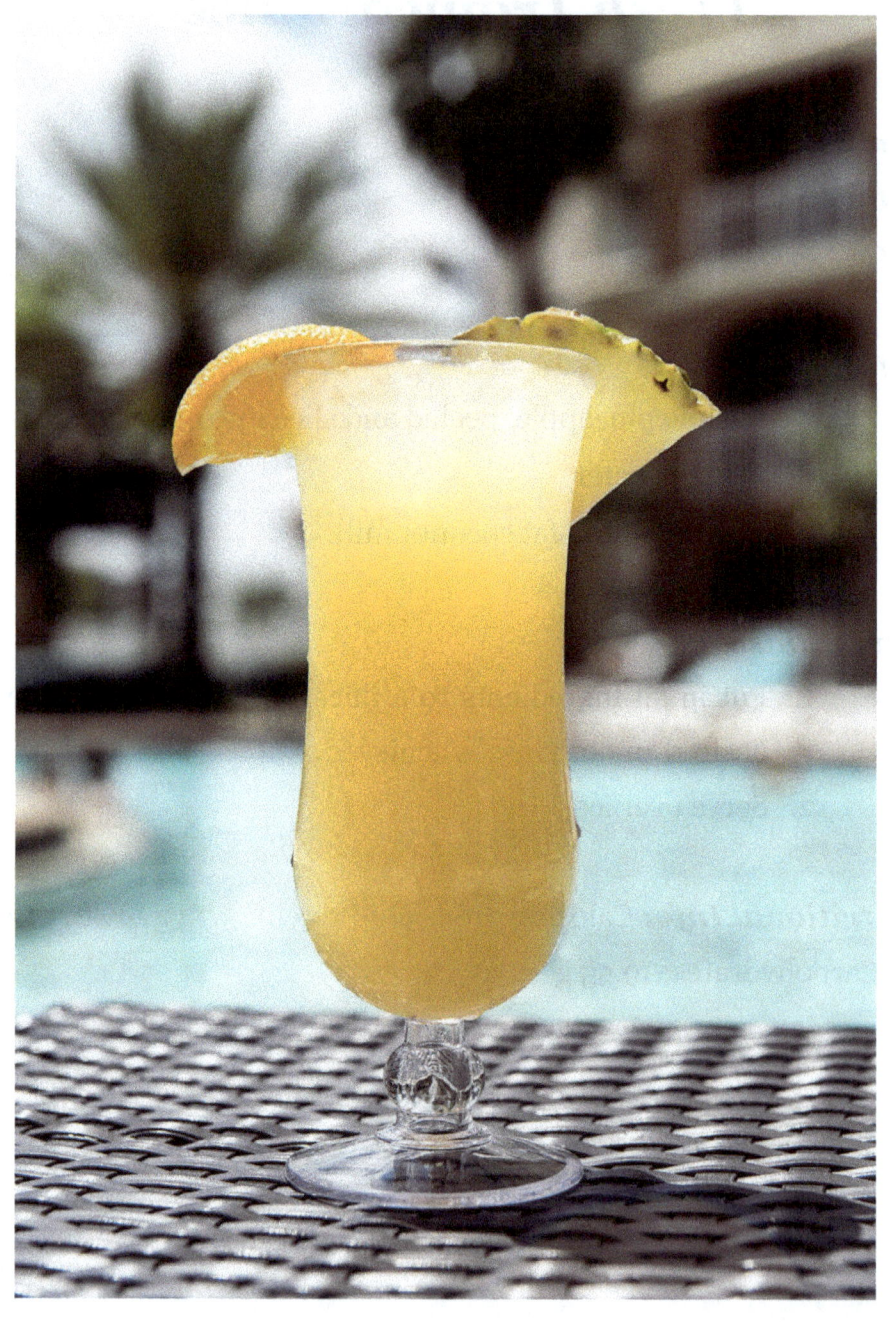

Ginger Ale

Time To Prepare: five minutes
Time to Cook: thirty minutes
Yield: Servings 4

Ingredients:

- 1 pound fresh ginger, unpeeled, diced
- 1 quart carbonated water
- 1 tbsp. honey
- Ice for serving
- Juice and rind of 2 lemons
- Lime wedges

Directions:

1. Put ginger and lemon juice in a food processor. Pulse to smooth consistency.
2. Move puree to the instant pot. Mix in honey.
3. Put in lemon peel to the instant pot.
4. Secure the lid. Cook on HIGH pressure thirty minutes.
5. When done, depressurize naturally. Strain and chill.
6. Serve over ice.

Nutritional Info: Calories: 108 ‖ Fat: 0g ‖ Carbohydrates: 28g ‖ Protein: 0g

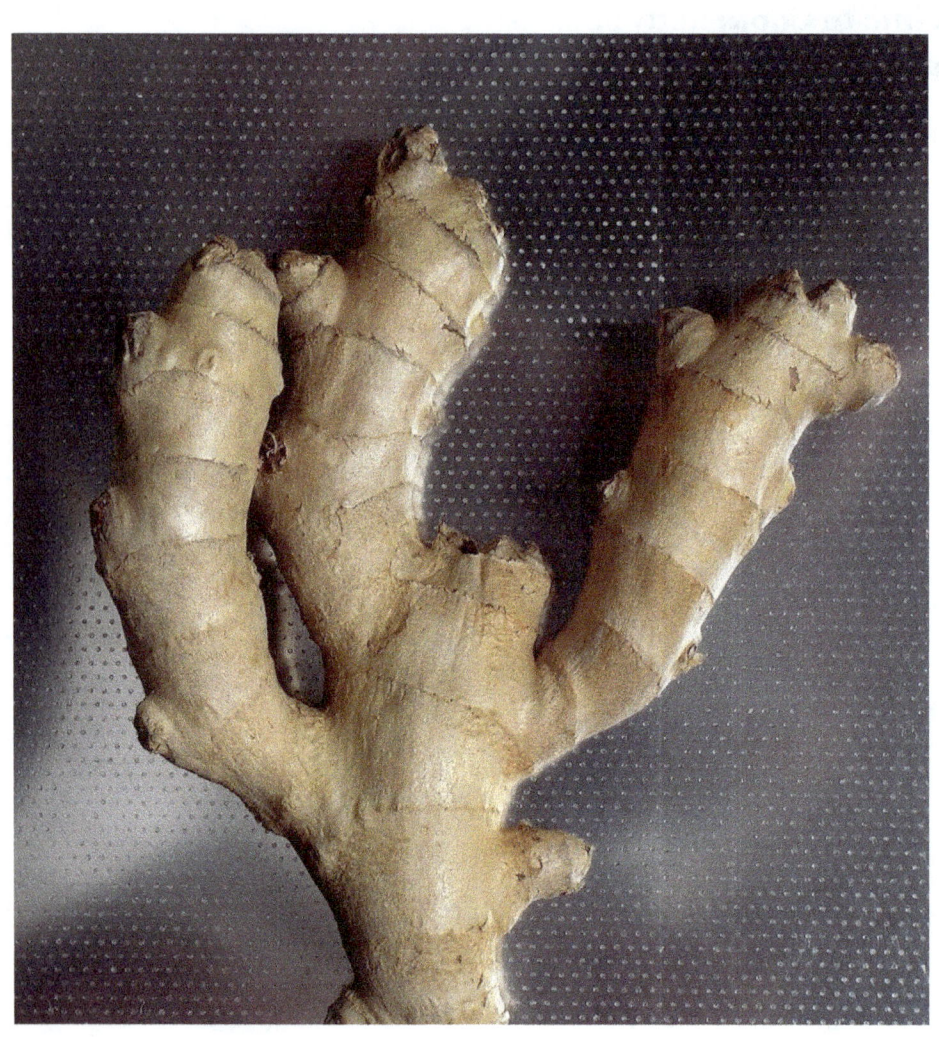

Ginger, Carrot, and Turmeric Smoothie

Time To Prepare: five minutes

Time to Cook: 0 minutes

Yield: Servings 2

Ingredients:

- ½ cup Mango, fresh or frozen chunks
- 1 big Carrot, peeled and chopped
- 1 cup Coconut water
- 1 Orange, peeled and separated
- 1 tbsp. Hemp seeds, raw, shelled
- 1 tsp. Ginger, ground
- 1 tsp. Turmeric, ground
- 1/8 tsp. Cayenne pepper

Directions:

Puree all of the ingredients with one-half cup of ice until the desired smoothness is achieved and drink instantly.

Nutritional Info: Calories 250 ‖ 35 grams sugar ‖ 4.5 grams fat ‖ 7 grams fiber ‖ 48 grams carbs ‖ 6 grams protein

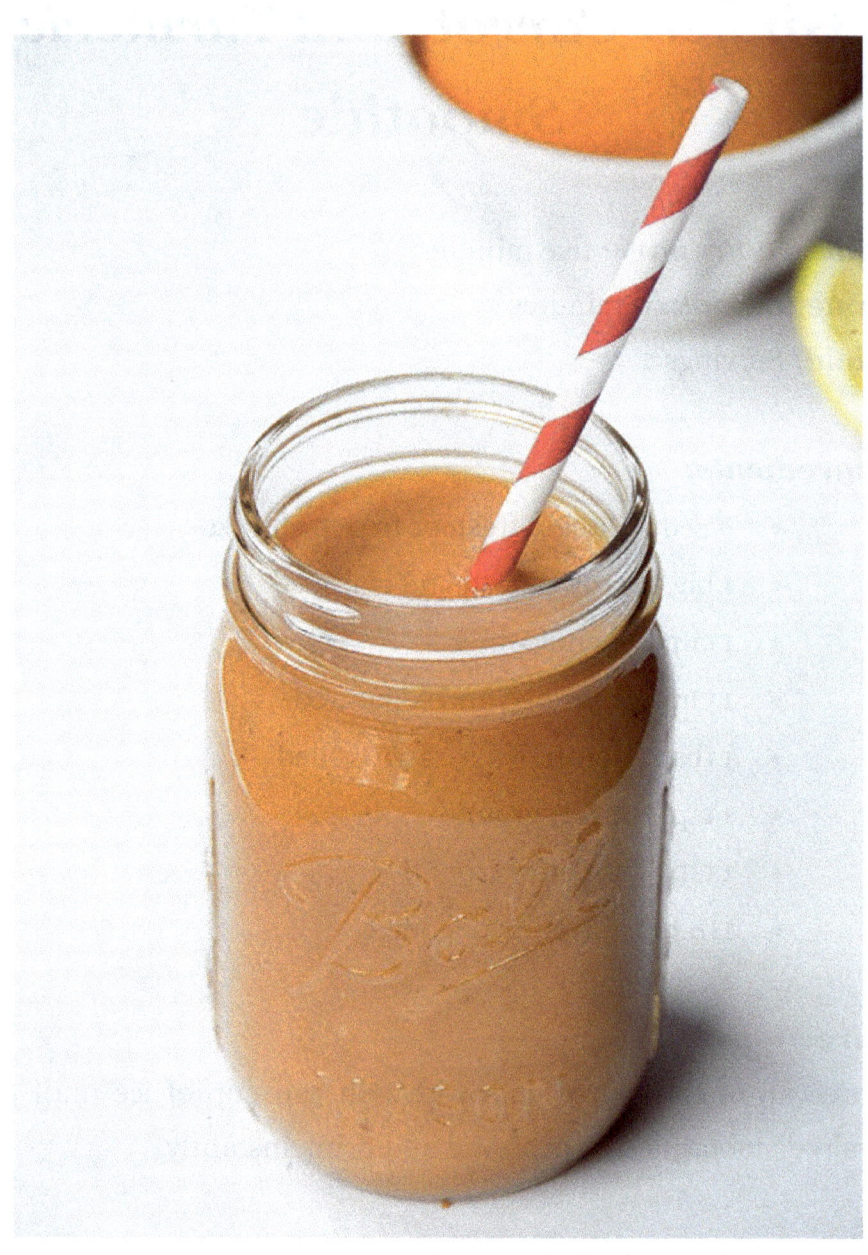

Golden Chai Latte

Time To Prepare: five minutes
Time to Cook: ten minutes
Yield: Servings 2

Ingredients:
- ¼ teaspoon ground cinnamon
- ½ cup water
- ½ tablespoon maple syrup
- ½ tablespoon turmeric powder
- 1 ¼ cups cashew milk or any other non-dairy milk of your choice
- 1 teaspoon loose leaf chai tea
- 1/8 teaspoon ground nutmeg
- A pinch ground cardamom

Directions:
1. Put in water and 1-cup milk into a deep cooking pan. Put the deep cooking pan on moderate heat.
2. Put in chai leaves in a tea strainer (the type that that has a lid and you can close). Lower the strainer in the deep cooking pan. Put in spices.

3. When it just comes to a light boil, remove the heat. Allow it to cool for five minutes. Take out the tea strainer and discard the leaves.
4. Put in maple syrup and stir.
5. Pour into glasses. Sprinkle remaining cashew milk on top. Decorate using cinnamon and nutmeg before you serve.

Nutritional Info: Calories: 142 kcal ‖ Protein: 8.59 g ‖ Fat: 6.26 g ‖ Carbohydrates: 13.3 g

SIDES

Goat Cheese Salad

Time To Prepare: fifteen minutes
Time to Cook: thirty minutes
Yield: Servings 4

Ingredients:

- ½ cup of walnuts
- ½ head of escarole (medium), torn
- 1 bunch of trimmed and torn arugula
- 1/3 cup extra virgin olive oil
- 2 bunches of medium beets (~1 ½ lbs.) with trimmed tops
- 2 tbsp. of red wine vinegar
- 4 oz. crumbled of goat cheese (aged cheese is preferred)
- Kosher salt + freshly ground black pepper

Directions:

1. Place the beets in water in a deep cooking pan and apply salt as seasoning. Now, boil them using high heat for approximately twenty minutes or until they're

soft. Peel them off when they're cool using your fingers or use a knife.
2. To taste, whisk the vinegar with salt and pepper in a big container. Then mix in the olive oil for the dressing. Toss the beets with the dressing, so they're uniformly coated and marinate them for approximately fifteen minutes – 2 hours.
3. Set the oven to 350F. Bring the nuts on a baking sheet and toast them for approximately 8 minutes (stirring them once) until they turn golden brown. Let them cool.
4. Mix and toss the escarole and arugula with the beets and put them in four plates. Put in the walnuts and goat cheese as toppings before you serve.
5. Enjoy!

Nutritional Info: ‖ Calories: 285 kcal ‖ Protein: 11.85 g ‖ Fat: 25.79 g ‖ Carbohydrates: 2.01 g

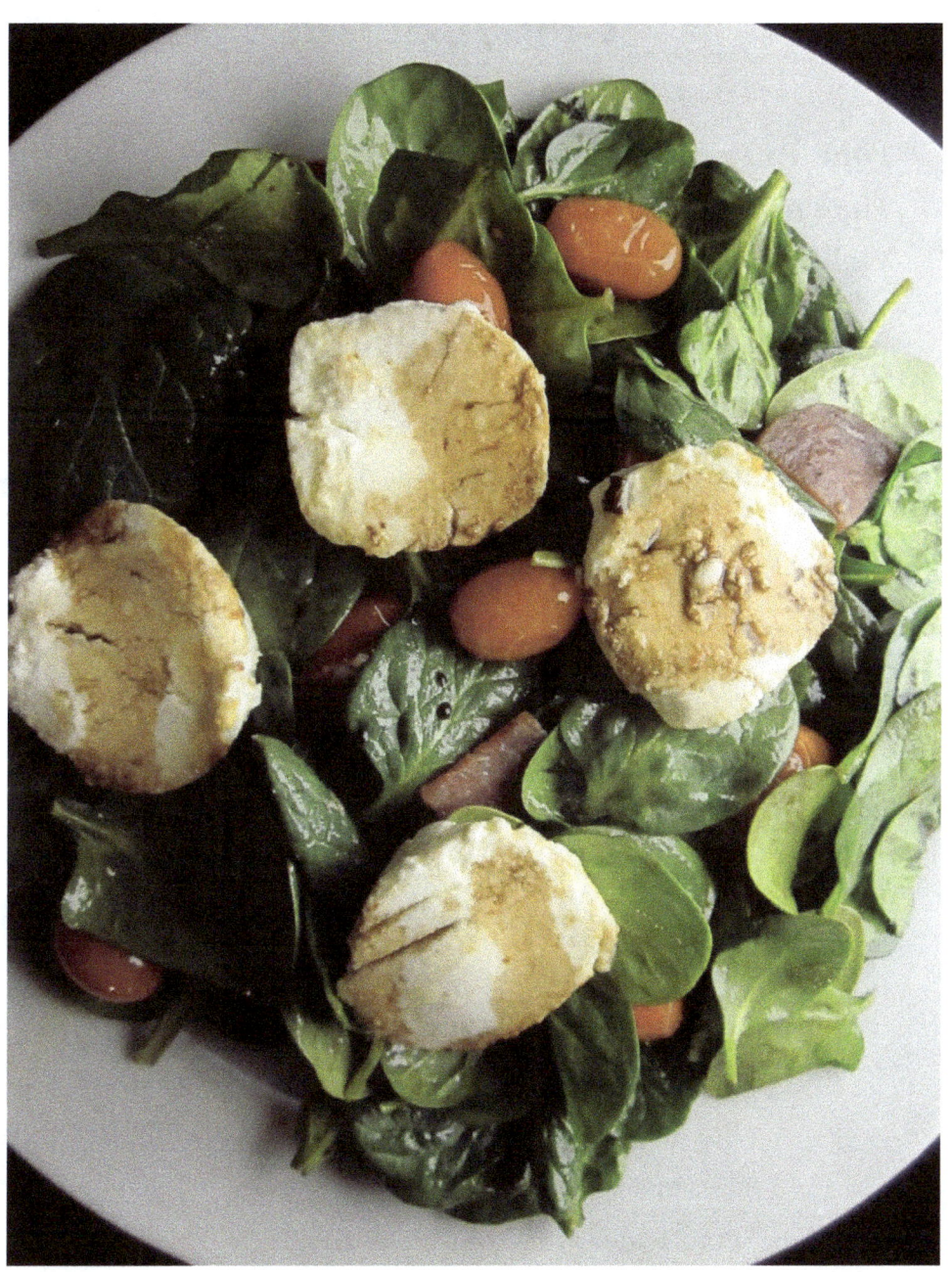

Green Beans

Time To Prepare: five minutes
Time to Cook: ten minutes
Yield: Servings 5

Ingredients:

- ½ teaspoon kosher salt
- ½ teaspoon of red pepper flakes
- 1½ lbs. green beans, trimmed
- 2 garlic cloves, minced
- 2 tablespoons of extra-virgin olive oil
- 2 tablespoons of water

Directions:

1. Heat oil in a frying pan on medium temperature.
2. Include the pepper flake. Stir to coat in the olive oil.
3. Include the green beans. Cook for seven minutes.
4. Stir frequently. The beans must be brown in some areas.
5. Put in the salt and garlic. Cook for a minute, while stirring.
6. Pour water and cover instantly.
7. Cook covered for 1 more minute.

Nutritional Info: Calories 82 ‖ Carbohydrates: 6g ‖ Total Fat: 6g ‖ Protein: 1g ‖ Fiber: 2g ‖ Sugar: 0g ‖ Sodium: 230mg

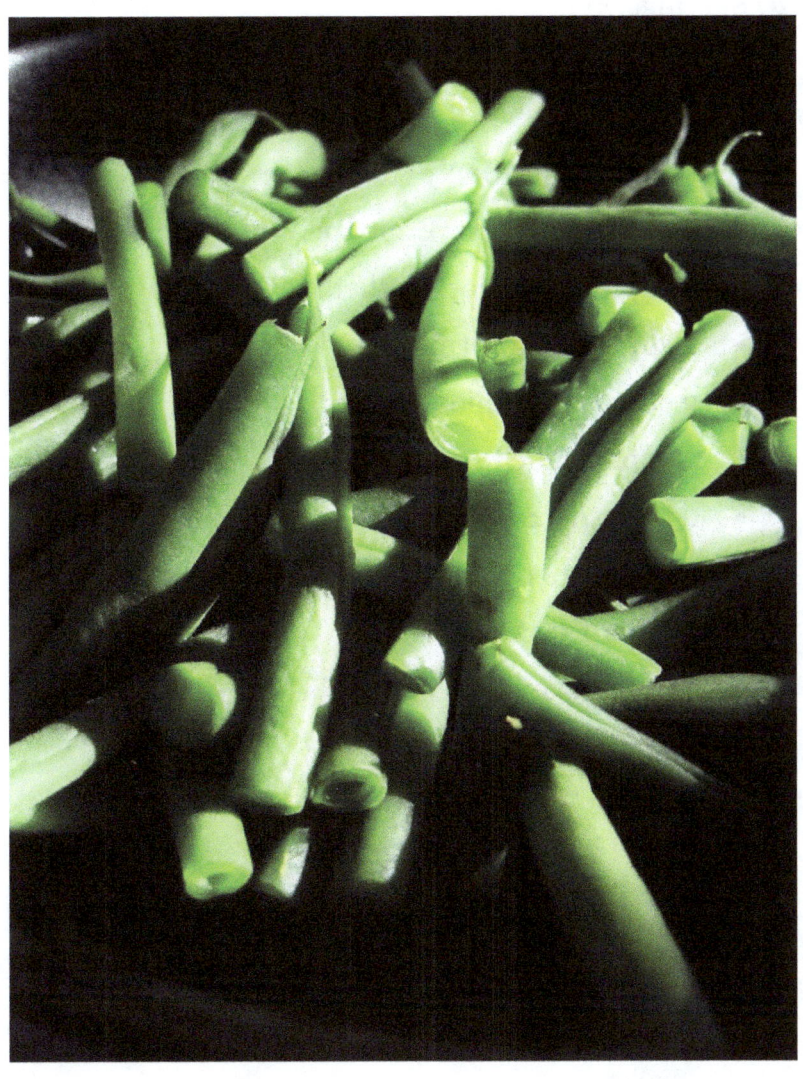

Green, Red and Yellow Rice

Time To Prepare: five minutes
Time to Cook: fifteen minutes
Yield: Servings 10

Ingredients:

- ¼ cup garlic, finely chopped
- 1 cup fresh cilantro, chopped
- 2 cups brown rice, washed
- 2 cups frozen corn, thawed
- 2 cups green onions, chopped
- 2 cups red bell pepper, chopped
- 2 tablespoons olive oil
- Cayenne pepper to taste
- Pepper to taste
- Salt to taste

Directions:

1. Put a big deep cooking pan on moderate heat. Put in 4 cups water and brown rice and cook in accordance with the instructions on the package. Once cooked, cover and save for later.

2. Put a big frying pan on moderate heat. Put in oil. When the oil is heated, put in garlic and sauté for approximately one minute until aromatic.
3. Put in corn, red bell pepper, green onion, salt, pepper and cayenne pepper and sauté for at least two minutes.
4. Put in rice and cilantro. Mix thoroughly and heat meticulously.
5. Serve.

Nutritional Info: ‖ Calories: 89 kcal ‖ Protein: 2.41 g ‖ Fat: 4.01 g ‖ Carbohydrates: 11.26 g

Hot Pink Coconut Slaw

Time To Prepare: five minutes
Time to Cook: 0 minutes
Yield: Servings 3

Ingredients:

- ¼ cup fresh cilantro, chopped
- ¼ teaspoon salt
- ½ cup big coconut flakes, unsweetened or shredded coconut, unsweetened
- ½ cup radish, thinly cut or shredded carrots
- ½ small jalapeño, deseeded, discard membranes, chopped
- ½ tablespoon honey or maple syrup
- 1 cup red onion, thinly cut
- 1 tablespoon olive oil
- 2 cups purple cabbage, thinly cut
- 2 tablespoons apple cider vinegar
- 2 tablespoons lime juice

Directions:
1. Combine all ingredients into a container and toss thoroughly. Cover and set aside for about forty minutes.
2. Toss thoroughly before you serve.

Nutritional Info: ‖ Calories: 179 kcal ‖ Protein: 3.92 g ‖ Fat: 10.64 g ‖ Carbohydrates: 18.53 g

SAUCES AND DRESSINGS

Creamy Raspberry Vinaigrette

Time To Prepare: ten minutes
Time to Cook: 0 minutes
Yield: Servings 2-4

Ingredients:

- ½ cup of raspberries
- 1 tbsp. of Dijon mustard
- 1 tbsp. of Greek yogurt
- 1/3 cup of extra-virgin olive oil
- 2 tbsp. of honey or maple syrup
- 2 tbsp. of raspberry vinegar

Directions:

1. Put all together the ingredients apart from the oil into a blender, in accordance with the ordered list. Cover and blend for ten seconds, by slowly increasing the speed.
2. After 10 seconds, reduce the speed and progressively put in the oil into the mixture. Keep the speed at a

stable pace until all of the oil has been poured in. Blend until blended.
3. Store in a mason jar then place in your fridge for maximum 5 days. Serve with a vegetable or fruit salad.

Nutritional Info: ‖ Calories: 151 kcal ‖ Protein: 2.22 g ‖ Fat: 9.47 g ‖ Carbohydrates: 14.65 g

Creamy Siamese Dressing

Time To Prepare: ten minutes
Time to Cook: 0 minutes
Yield: Servings 2-4

Ingredients:

- ¼ cup of non-dairy milk (e.g., almond, rice, soymilk)
- ¼ cup of unsweetened peanut sauce
- 1 cup of mayonnaise
- 1 tbsp. of honey or maple syrup
- 1 tbsps. freshly chopped cilantro
- 2 tbsp. of unsalted peanuts
- 2 tbsp. rice vinegar

Directions:

1. Put all ingredients apart from the cilantro and peanuts into a blender and blend until the desired smoothness is achieved and creamy. Next, put in in the cilantro and peanuts and pulse the blender a few times until completely crushed and well blended. Put in a mason jar and bring it in your fridge.
2. Serve with a garden salad, pasta or as a dipping sauce.

Nutritional Info: ∥ Calories: 525 kcal ∥ Protein: 18.14 g ∥ Fat: 45.55 g ∥ Carbohydrates: 11.01 g

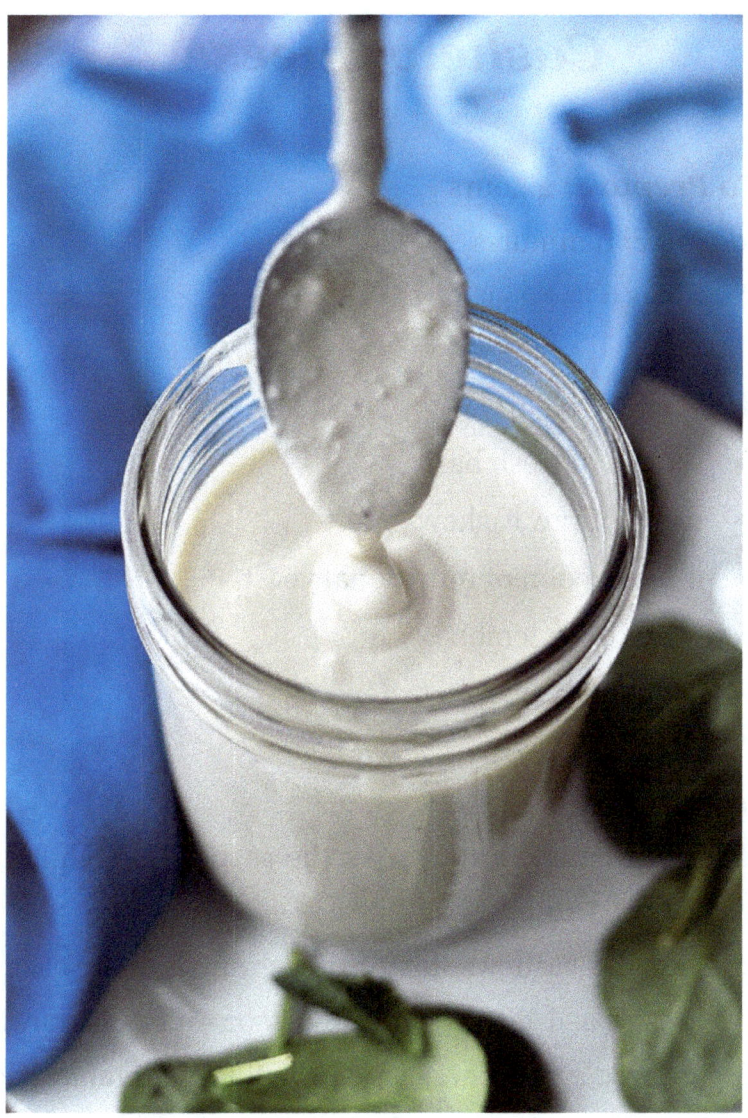

SNACKS

Cashew Cheese

Time To Prepare: 2 hours
Time to Cook: 0 minutes
Yield: Servings 6

Ingredients:

- ¼ cup of fresh basil
- 1 cup of raw cashews
- 1 tablespoon of nutritional yeast
- Juice of ½ lemon
- Salt and pepper to taste

Directions:

1. In a1 cup of water, soak the cashew for minimum 2 hours. Drain.
2. Put the cashews, lemon juice, nutritional yeast, and fresh basil into a food processor and pulse until the desired smoothness is achieved. Put in 1 tablespoon of water at a time to make it creamy, but not runny.
3. Flavor it with pepper and salt, then spread it on gluten-free bread or toast.

4. Store in an airtight jar in your fridge.

Nutritional Info: ‖ Total Carbohydrates: 126g ‖ Fiber: 1g ‖ Net Carbohydrates: ‖ Protein: 4g ‖ Total Fat: 10g ‖ Calories: 126

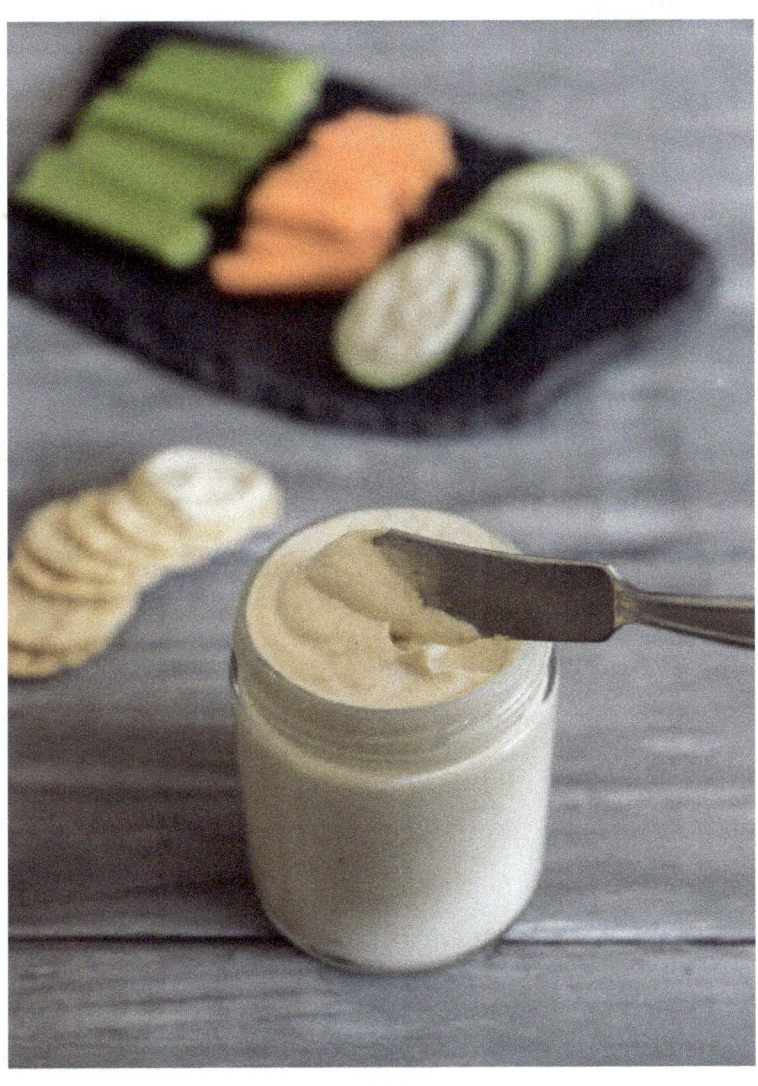

Cauliflower Snacks

Time To Prepare: ten minutes
Time to Cook: 60 minutes
Yield: Servings 4

Ingredients:

- 1 head of cauliflower
- 1 teaspoon salt
- 4 tablespoons extra virgin olive oil

Directions:

1. Set the oven to 425F, then prepare two cookie sheets by lining them using parchment paper.
2. Trim off the cauliflower florets and discard the core. Chop the florets into golf-ball-sized pieces.
3. Put the cauliflower in a container, and pour olive oil over them and drizzle with salt. Mix to coat. Spread in a single layer, not touching.
4. Roast approximately 1 hour flipping the cauliflower three to four times until a golden-brown color is achieved. Serve warm.

Nutritional Info: ‖ Calories: 91 kcal ‖ Protein: 2.93 g ‖ Fat: 7.7 g ‖ Carbohydrates: 3.29 g

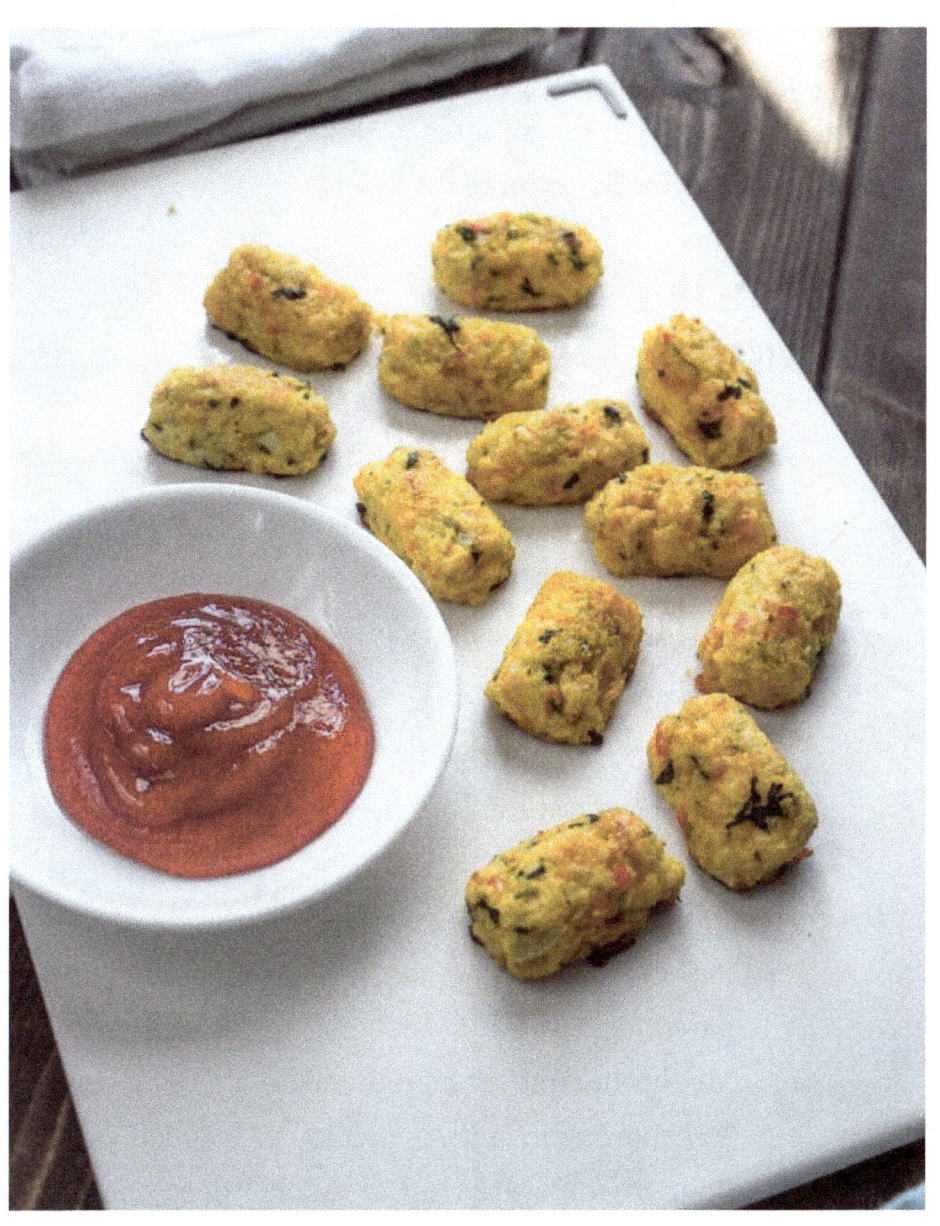

Cereal Chia Chips

Time To Prepare: ten minutes
Time to Cook: thirty minutes
Yield: Servings 10

Ingredients:

- ¼-cup rolled oats, gluten-free
- ½-cup maple syrup
- ½-cup white quinoa, uncooked
- ¾-cup pecans, chopped
- 2-Tbsps chia seeds
- 2-Tbsps coconut oil
- 2-Tbsps coconut sugar
- A pinch of sea salt (not necessary)

Directions:

1. Preheat the oven to 325°F. Coat a baking pan using parchment paper.
2. Mix in the first six ingredients in a mixing container. Mix thoroughly until meticulously blended. Set aside.
3. Pour the oil and syrup in a small deep cooking pan placed on moderate to low heat. Heat the mixture for about three minutes, stirring once in a while.

4. Fold in the dry ingredients; stir thoroughly to coat completely.
5. Pour the mixture in the baking pan, and spread to a uniform layer using a spoon.
6. Place the pan in your oven. Bake for fifteen minutes. Turn the pan around to cook uniformly. Bake for 8-ten minutes until the mixture turns golden brown.
7. Allow cooling completely before breaking the chips into bite-size pieces.

Nutritional Info: ‖ Calories: 157 ‖ Fat: 5.2g ‖ Protein: 7.8g S ‖ Sodium: 25mg ‖ Total Carbohydrates: 22.1g ‖ Fiber: 2.5g ‖ Net Carbohydrates: 19.6g

Chewy Blackberry Leather

Time To Prepare: fifteen minutes
Time to Cook: 5-6 hours
Yield: Servings 8

Ingredients:

- ¼ cup of raw honey
- 1 tbsp. of fresh mint leaves
- 1 tsp. of ground cinnamon
- 1/8 tsp. of fresh lemon juice
- 2 cups of fresh blackberries

Directions:

1. Set the oven to 170F. Coat baking sheet using parchment paper.
2. Use a food processor to put all ingredients and pulse till smooth.
3. Take the mixture onto the readied baking sheet and, using the backside of a spoon, smooth the top.
4. Bake for approximately 5-6 hours.
5. Chop the leather into equal-sized strips.
6. Now, roll each rectangle to make fruit rolls.

Nutritional Info: ‖ Calories: 49 ‖ Fat: 0.2g ‖ Carbohydrates: 12.5g ‖ Protein: 0.6g ‖ Fiber: 2.1g

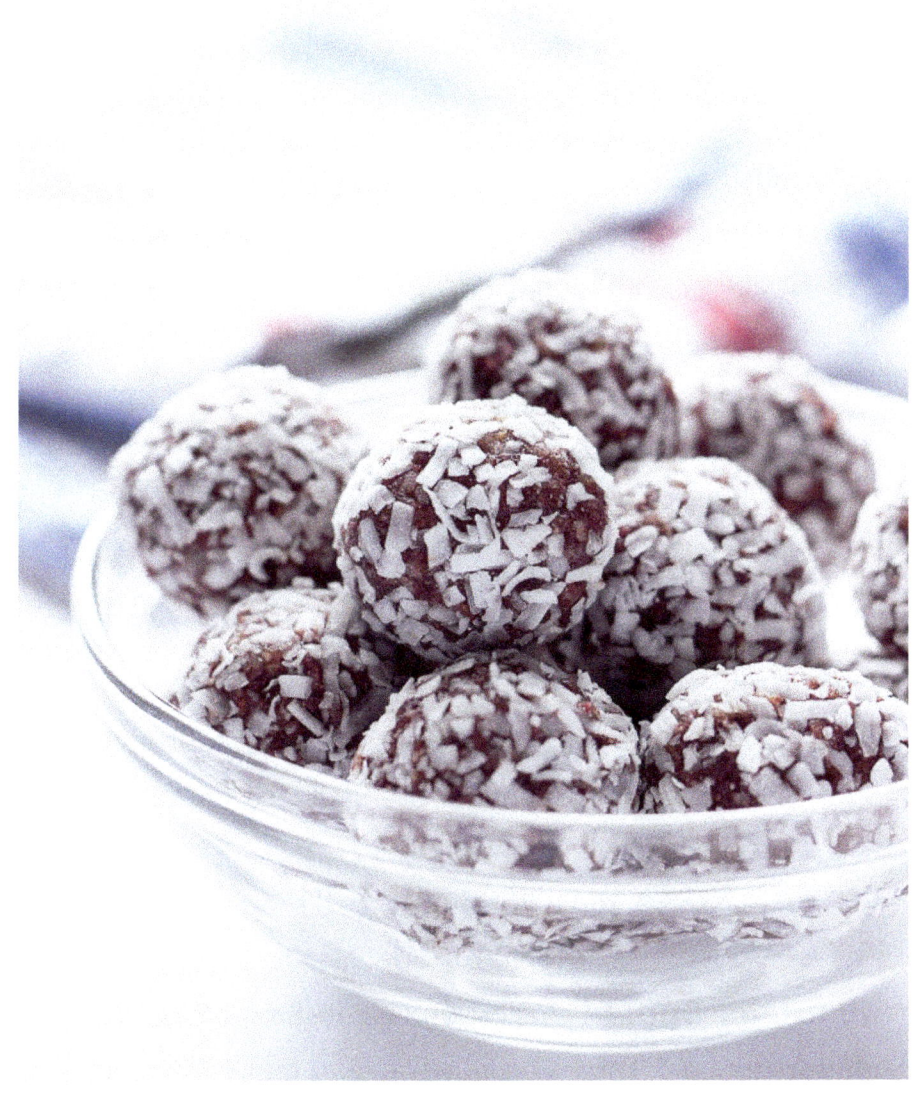

Chia Cashew Cream

Time To Prepare: 2 hours and five minutes
Time to Cook: 0 minutes
Yield: Servings 1

Ingredients:

- ¼-cup quinoa, cooked
- ¼-tsp vanilla powder
- ¾-cup cashew milk
- 2-Tbsps chia seeds
- 2-Tbsps hemp hearts
- 2-Tbsps maple syrup or a dash of liquid stevia
- A pinch of cinnamon

Directions:

1. Mix all the ingredients in a jar. Mix thoroughly until meticulously blended. Cover the jar and place in your fridge for about two hours.
2. To serve, top with your desired toppings.

Nutritional Info: ‖ Calories: 258 ‖ Fat: 8.6g ‖ Protein: 12.9g ‖ Sodium: 123mg ‖ Total Carbohydrates: 34.2g ‖ Fiber: 2g ‖ Net Carbohydrates: 32.2g

Coco Cherry Bake-less Bars

Time To Prepare: ten minutes
Time to Cook: 0 minutes
Yield: Servings 6

Ingredients:

- ¼-cup pure maple syrup
- ⅓-cup coconut, unsweetened and shredded
- ⅓-cup dried cherries or cranberries
- ⅓-cup ground flaxseed
- ½-cup almond butter
- 1-cup old-fashioned oats
- 1-Tbsp almond milk
- 1-Tbsp vanilla extract
- 3-scoops vanilla plant-based Protein powder

Directions:

1. Coat a loaf pan using parchment paper.
2. Mix in the first four ingredients in your blender. Blend until the mixture becomes powdery.
3. Move the mixture to a mixing container. Put in in all the rest of the ingredients. Mix thoroughly until meticulously blended.

4. Put the mixture in the pan, and press down onto a consistently flat surface.
5. Freeze for thirty minutes before cutting into six bars.

Nutritional Info: ‖ Calories: 193 ‖ Fat: 6.4g ‖ Protein: 9.6g ‖ Sodium: 200mg ‖ Total Carbohydrates: 27.1g ‖ Fiber: 3g ‖ Net Carbohydrates: 24.1g

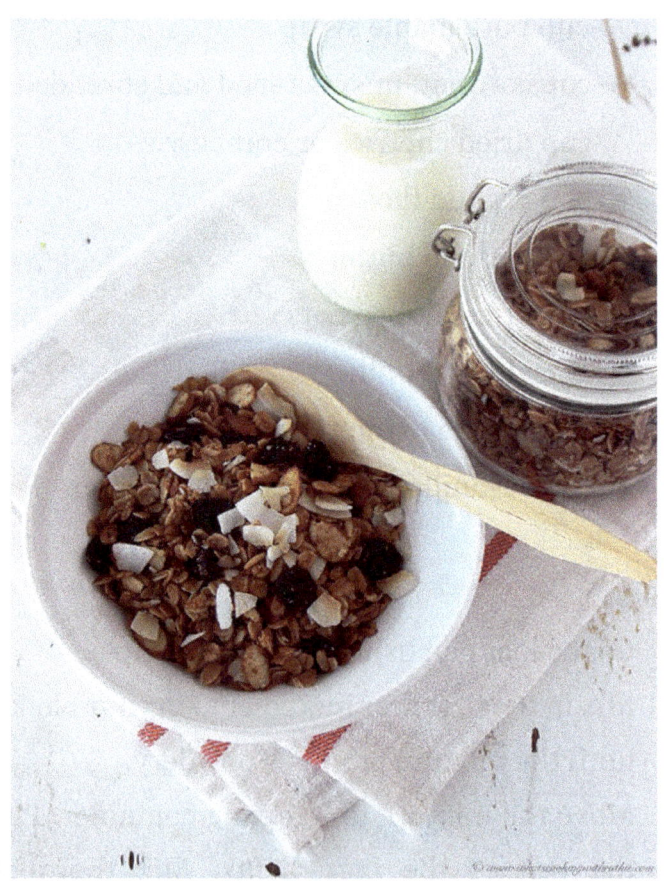

Coconut Porridge

Time To Prepare: twenty minutes
Time to Cook: ten minutes
Yield: Servings 2

Ingredients:

- 1 tbsp. coconut oil
- 1 tsp cinnamon
- 1 vanilla bean
- 2 cups oats
- 2 tbsp. maple syrup
- 2 tsp ginger
- 2 tsp turmeric
- 330ml vaporized coconut milk
- 750 ml of water
- Coconut milk
- Fresh, shredded coconut (for serving)

Directions:

1. Mix 750 ml water and turmeric in a container. Allow it to sit for about ten minutes.
2. Combine all ingredients apart from coconut milk and shredded coconut in a deep cooking pan.

3. Heat it on medium heat while stirring continuously, and cook for eight minutes.
4. Allow it to cool for about ten minutes.
5. Split into serving bowls.
6. Put in coconut milk and shredded coconut on top.
7. Put in some extra cinnamon to your taste.
8. Eat warm.

Nutritional Info: ‖ Calories: 417 kcal ‖ Protein: 20.63 g ‖ Fat: 16.8 g ‖ Carbohydrates: 83.03 g

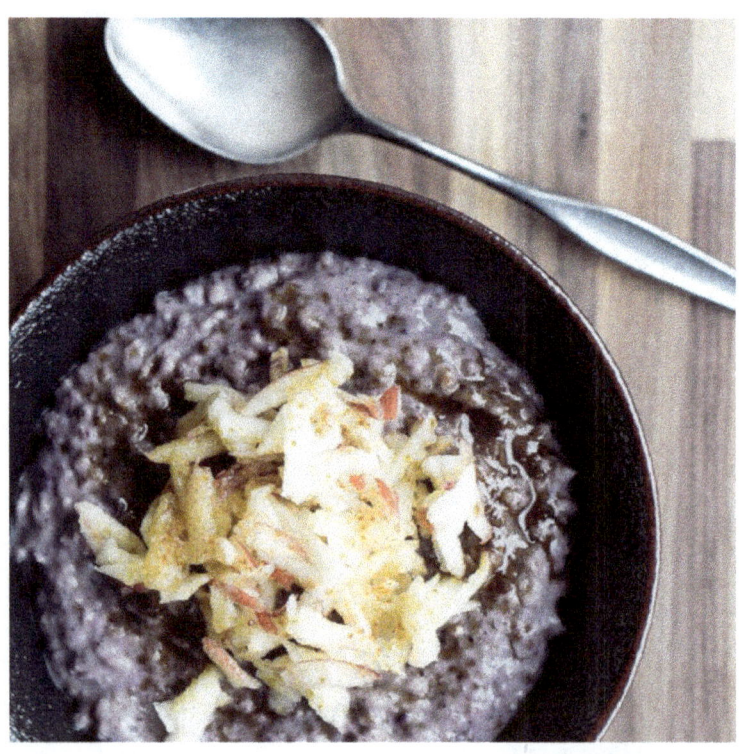

SOUPS AND STEWS

Creamy Leek Soup

Time To Prepare: two minutes
Time to Cook: 8 minutes
Yield: Servings 4

Ingredients:

- ½ cup heavy cream
- ½ cup Monterey-Jack cheese, shredded
- ½ cup tomato purée
- ½ pound chorizo, cut
- 1 bay leaf
- 1 cup leeks, chopped
- 1 green chili, deseeded and finely chopped
- 1 tablespoon sesame oil
- 2 chicken bouillon cubes
- 2 cloves garlic, minced
- 4 cups water

Directions:

1. Push the "Sauté" button to heat up your Instant Pot. Once hot, heat the oil and sauté the leeks until soft.

2. Now, mix in chorizo, garlic, and green chili; carry on cooking until aromatic. Next, put in water, tomato puree, heavy cream, bouillon cubes, and bay leaf.
3. Secure the lid. Choose "Manual" mode and High pressure; cook for about six minutes. Once cooking is complete, use a natural pressure release; cautiously remove the lid.
4. Next, press the "Sauté" button and put in the cheese; allow it to simmer until the cheese is melted and thoroughly heated.

Nutritional Info: 428 Calories ‖ 36g Fat ‖ 6.1g Total Carbs ‖ 18.9g Protein ‖ 2.1g Sugars

Creamy Parsnip Soup

Time To Prepare: twenty-five minutes
Time to Cook: 60 minutes
Yield: Servings 10

Ingredients:

- 1 big onion (diced)
- 1 cup whole milk
- 1 tablespoon brown sugar
- 1 tablespoon butter
- 1 tablespoon olive oil
- 1 teaspoon ground ginger
- ½ teaspoon ground allspice
- ½ teaspoon ground cardamom
- ½ teaspoon ground nutmeg
- 1/4 teaspoon cayenne pepper
- 2 pounds parsnips (peeled, cut)
- 3 carrots (peeled, cut)
- 3 cloves garlic (minced)
- 3 stalks celery (diced)
- 4 cups chicken stock
- Ground black pepper
- Salt

Directions:
1. Preheat your oven to 425 F.
2. Toss the parsnips and carrots with oil and seasoning in a container. Put them over a baking sheet.
3. Roast in oven until for half an hour
4. Cook the onion and celery in oil till golden brown, approximately seven minutes. Put in butter, brown sugar, garlic, and the parsnips and carrots, cooking for about ten minutes.
5. Season and stir. Put in the chicken stock to its boiling point until soft.
6. Puree the soup.
7. Put in milk and cream and simmer some more before you serve with seasoning.

Nutritional Info: Calories: 187 kcal ‖ Carbohydrates: 24 g ‖ Fat: 9 g ‖ Protein: 3 g

Creamy Pumpkin Puree Soup

Time To Prepare: ten minutes
Time to Cook: forty-five minutes
Yield: Servings 3

Ingredients:

- 1 cup Heavy Cream
- 1 cup Pumpkin puree
- 2 cups Chicken broth
- 2 tbsp. Olive oil
- 4-5 Garlic cloves
- Salt and black pepper to taste

Directions:

1. In the Instant Pot, put in all ingredients.
2. Secure the lid and cook for forty minutes on Meat/Stew mode on High. When ready, press Cancel and do a quick pressure release.
3. Move to a blender and blend thoroughly. Pour into serving bowls to serve.

Nutritional Info: Calories 465 ‖ Protein: 15.4g ‖ Carbs: 6.2g ‖ Fat: 43.5g

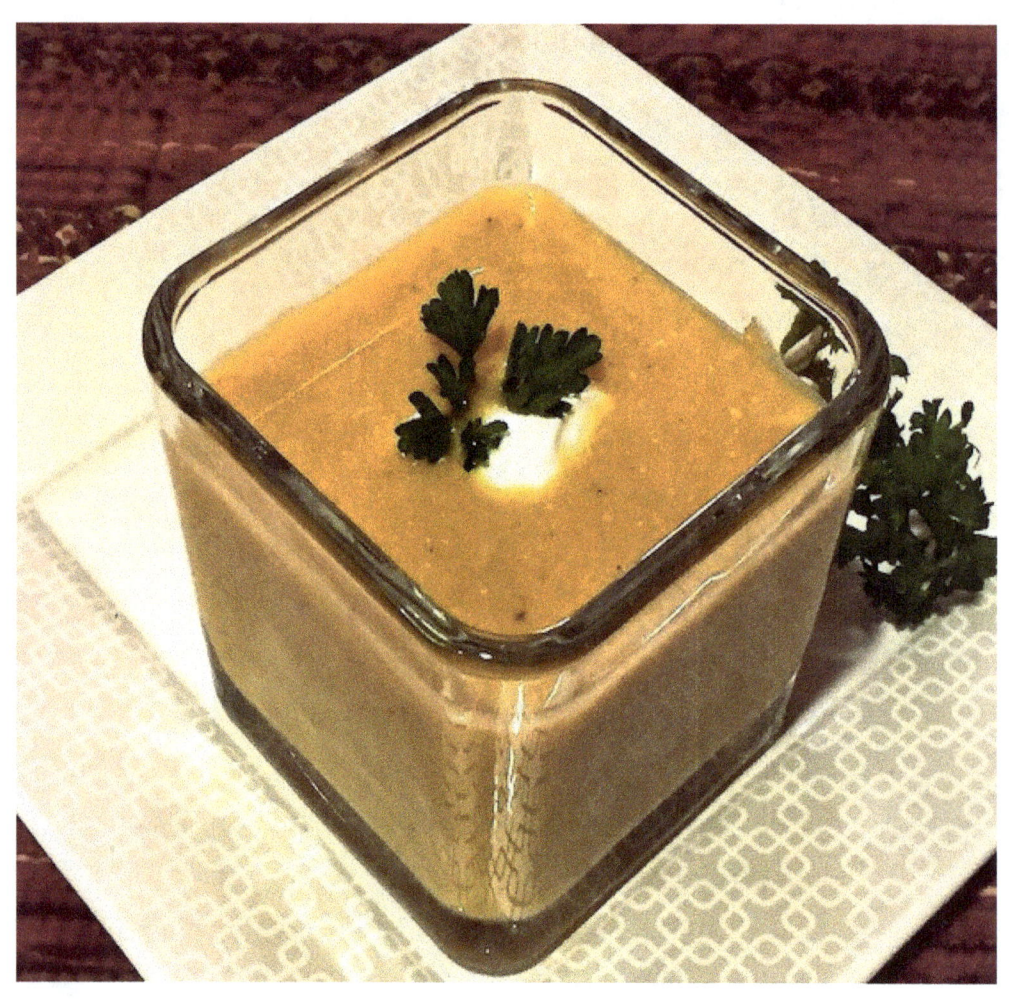

Creamy Turkey Soup

Time To Prepare: fifteen minutes
Time to Cook: 4 hours
Yield: Servings 7

Ingredients:

- 1 carrot, chopped
- 1 cup cream cheese
- 1 pound turkey breast, cubed
- 1 stalk celery, chopped
- 1 teaspoon freshly chopped rosemary
- 3 cloves garlic, chopped
- 5 cups chicken broth
- Salt & black pepper, to taste

Directions:

1. Put in all the ingredients minus the cream cheese to the base of a slow cooker.
2. Cook on high for 4 hours.
3. Mix in the cream cheese until well blended.

Nutritional Info: Calories: 216 ‖ Carbohydrates: 6g ‖ Fiber: 1g Net ‖ Carbohydrates: 5g ‖ Fat: 14g ‖ Protein: 17g

Creamy Turmeric Cauliflower Soup

Time To Prepare: ten minutes
Time to Cook: fifteen minutes
Yield: Servings 4

Ingredients:

- ¼ cup finely chopped fresh cilantro
- ¼ teaspoon freshly ground black pepper
- ¼ teaspoon ground cumin
- ½ teaspoon salt
- 1 (1¼-inch) piece fresh ginger, peeled and cut
- 1 cup full-fat coconut milk
- 1 garlic clove, peeled
- 1 leek, white part only, thinly cut
- 1½ teaspoons turmeric
- 2 tablespoons extra-virgin olive oil
- 3 cups cauliflower florets
- 3 cups vegetable broth

Directions:

1. In a large pot, heat the oil on high heat.

2. Put in the leek, and sauté until it just starts to brown, three to four minutes.
3. Put in the cauliflower, garlic, ginger, turmeric, salt, pepper, and cumin and sauté to lightly toast the spices, one to two minutes.
4. Pour the broth then bring to its boiling point.
5. Reduce the heat and cook until the cauliflower is soft about five minutes.
6. Use an immersion blender to purée the soup in the pot until the desired smoothness is achieved.
7. Stir in the coconut milk and cilantro, heat through, before you serve.

Nutritional Info: Calories: 264 ‖ Total Fat: 23g ‖ Total Carbohydrates: 12g ‖ Sugar: 5g ‖ Fiber: 4g ‖ Protein: 7g ‖ Sodium: 900mg

Crock-Pot Turkey Taco Soup

Time To Prepare: ten minutes
Time to Cook: 4 hours
Yield: Servings 6

Ingredients:

- 1 cup canned diced tomatoes (no sugar added)
- 1 cup whipped cream cheese
- 1 pound ground turkey
- 1 tablespoon chili powder
- 1 teaspoon cumin
- 1 teaspoon garlic powder
- 1 teaspoon onion powder
- 1 yellow onion, chopped
- 5 cups chicken bone broth (you can also use regular chicken broth)

Directions:

1. Put in all the ingredients to the base of a Crock-Pot minus the cream cheese and cover with the chicken broth.
2. Set on high and cook for 4 hours putting in in the cream cheese at the 3.5 hour mark.

3. Stir thoroughly before you serve.

Nutritional Info: Calories: 335‖ Carbohydrates: 6g‖ Fiber: 1gNet ‖ Carbohydrates: 5g‖ Fat: 23g‖ Protein: 28g

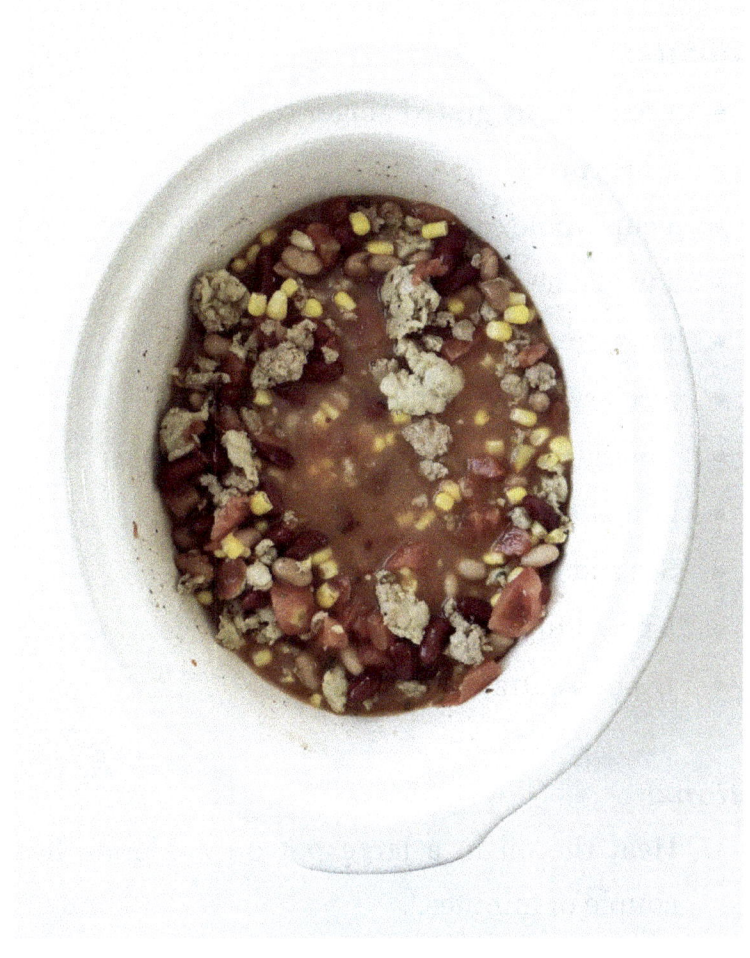

Detox Cabbage Soup

Time To Prepare: ten minutes
Time to Cook: thirty-five minutes
Yield: Servings 4

Ingredients:

- 1 tbs. freshly grated ginger root
- 2 big carrot
- 1 cup whole canned tomatoes with juice
- 1 whole head of cabbage
- 1 tbs. freshly grated turmeric root
- 3 celery stalks with leaves
- Enough water to immerse the vegetables
- 2 medium Russet potatoes
- Sea salt & black pepper to taste
- ½ medium onion
- 1/4 cup extra virgin olive oil

Directions:

1. Heat the oil in a large pot on moderate heat for a couple of minutes.

2. Put in the celery, onions, ginger, carrots & turmeric, then sauté on medium until translucent. Sprinkle with salt & pepper to taste.
3. With the heat still on moderate, dice the potatoes & generally slash the cabbage at that point put in to the pot alongside the whole tomatoes & juice.
4. While they cook, break separated the tomatoes using a fork or blade. Fill the pot with sufficient water to simply cover the cabbage.
5. Cover with a top & heat to the point of boiling. When bubbling, evacuate the top & cook for around thirty minutes or until the potatoes & cabbage are fork delicate. Put in the ice chest for as long as 5 days & in the cooler for as long as three months.

Nutritional Info: Calories: 359 kcal ‖ Protein: 10.85 g ‖ Fat: 12.68 g ‖ Carbohydrates: 54.94 g

Fennel and Pear Soup

Time To Prepare: fifteen minutes
Time to Cook: twenty minutes
Yield: Servings 4

Ingredients:

- ⅛ Teaspoon ground nutmeg
- ¼ cup freshly squeezed lemon juice
- ¼ cup honey
- ¼ teaspoon freshly ground black pepper
- 1 teaspoon finely chopped fresh tarragon
- 1 teaspoon salt
- 2 fennel bulbs, trimmed and slice into ½-inch dice
- 2 shallots, halved
- 2 tablespoons extra-virgin olive oil
- 4 cups vegetable broth
- 4 pears, cored and slice into ½-inch dice

Directions:

1. In a large pot, heat the oil on high heat.
2. Put in the pears, fennel, and shallots, and sauté until the pears and fennel barely start to brown, approximately five minutes.

3. Pour the broth, then bring to its boiling point.
4. Reduce the heat to a simmer, then cook, once in a while stirring, until the fennel is soft, 5 to 8 minutes.
5. Stir in the lemon juice, honey, salt, pepper, and nutmeg.
6. Use an immersion blender to purée the soup in the pot until the desired smoothness is achieved.
7. Drizzle with the tarragon before you serve.

Nutritional Info: Calories: 328 ‖ Total Fat: 9g ‖ Total Carbohydrates: 60g ‖ Sugar: 39g ‖ Fiber: 10g ‖ Protein: 7g ‖ Sodium: 1413mg

French Caramelized Onion Soup

Time To Prepare: five minutes
Time to Cook: ten minutes
Yield: Servings 4

Ingredients:

- ½ stick butter, softened
- 4 cups chicken stock
- ½ teaspoon dried basil
- Kosher salt and ground black pepper, to taste
- ½ cup Swiss cheese, freshly grated
- 3/4 pound yellow onions, cut

Directions:

1. Push the "Sauté" button to heat up your Instant Pot. Once hot, melt the butter and sauté the onions until caramelized and soft.
2. Put in chicken stock, basil, salt, and black pepper.
3. Secure the lid. Choose "Manual" mode and High pressure; cook for about ten minutes. Once cooking is complete, use a quick pressure release; cautiously remove the lid.
4. Ladle the soup into separate bowls and top with grated cheese. Enjoy!

Nutritional Info: 228 Calories ‖ 18g Fat ‖ 5.3g Total Carbs ‖ 10.5g Protein ‖ 3.5g Sugars

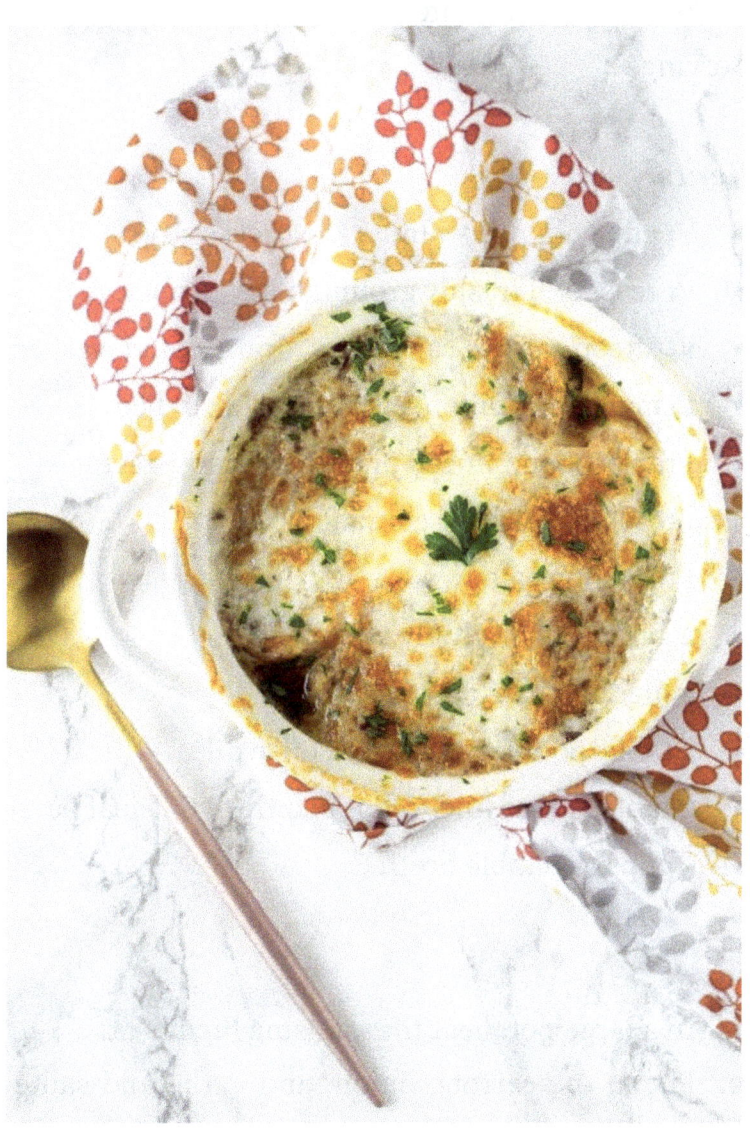

Garlic and Lentil Soup

Time To Prepare: fifteen minutes
Time to Cook: fifteen minutes
Yield: Servings 4

Ingredients:

- ¼ cup chopped walnuts (not necessary)
- ¼ teaspoon freshly ground black pepper
- 1 (fifteen-ounce) can lentils, drained and washed
- 1 small white onion, cut into ¼-inch dice
- 1 tablespoon minced or grated orange zest
- 1 teaspoon ground cinnamon
- 1 teaspoon salt
- 2 garlic cloves, thinly cut
- 2 medium carrots, thinly cut
- 2 tablespoons extra-virgin olive oil
- 2 tablespoons finely chopped fresh flat-leaf parsley
- 3 cups vegetable broth

Directions:

1. In a large pot, heat the oil using high heat.
2. Put in the carrots, onion, and garlic and sauté until tender, five to seven minutes.

3. Place the cinnamon, salt, and pepper and stir to uniformly coat the vegetables, one to two minutes.
4. Pour the broth then bring to its boiling point.
5. Reduce the heat to a simmer, put in the lentils and cook until they are thoroughly heated about one minute.
6. Mix in the orange zest and serve, sprinkled with the walnuts (if using) and parsley.

Nutritional Info: Calories: 201 ‖ Total Fat: 8g ‖ Total Carbohydrates 22g ‖ Sugar: 4g ‖ Fiber: 8g ‖ Protein: 11g ‖ Sodium: 1178mg

DESSERTS

Chocolate Mousse

Time To Prepare: 10 Minutes
Time to Cook: 0 Minute
Yield: Servings 4

Ingredients:

- 1 teaspoon of vanilla extract
- 3 tablespoons of Agave Nectar
- 4 tablespoons of cocoa
- Coconut cream scraped from the upper side of 2 pieces of 13.5-ounce chilled cans of full-fat coconut milk

Directions:

1. Take a big container and scoop out the thick coconut cream from the can to the container
2. Put in nectar, vanilla extract and cocoa to the container
3. Beat it well using an electric mixer, beginning from low and going to moderate until a foamy texture appears

4. Split the mix uniformly amongst ramekins and chill to your desired level of cold
5. Enjoy!

Nutritional Info: ‖ Calories: 134 Cal ‖ Fat: 3.8 g ‖ Carbohydrates: 16 g ‖ Protein: 3.8 g

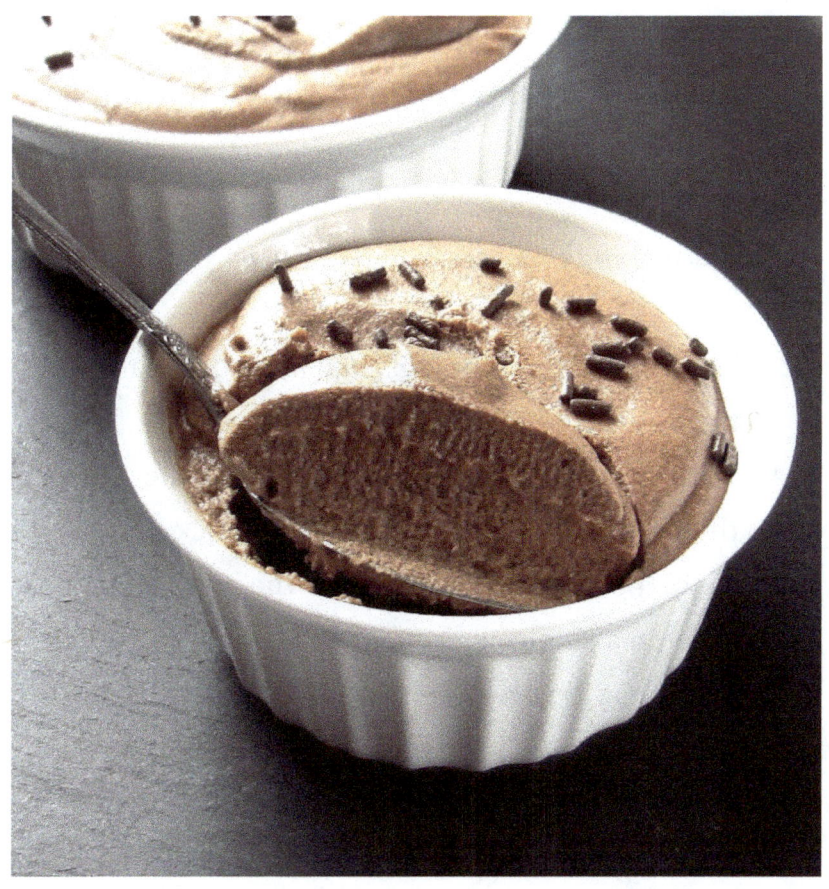

Cinnamon Apple Chips

Time To Prepare: 10 Minutes
Time to Cook: 2 Hours
Yield: Servings 3

Ingredients:

- ¾ tsp. Cinnamon, grounded
- 3 Honey crisp Apple, big & sweet

Directions:

1. For making this dessert fare, preheat your oven to 200 °F.
2. Next, keep a parchment paper-lined baking sheet in the center and lower rack.
3. With the help of an apple corer, core the apples and then slice the apples into 1/8-inch-thick rounds.
4. Next, position the apples in the preheated baking sheet in a single layer.
5. After this, drizzle the cinnamon over the apples.
6. Once sprinkled, bake them for an hour.
7. Take away the baking sheet and then switch their position.
8. Bake them for another one to 1 ½ hour or until the chips are crunchy.

9. To finish, once they are crisp in accordance with your liking, remove the apple chips from the oven.
10. Let the chips cool for one hour before you serve.

Nutritional Info: ‖ Calories: 96Kcal ‖ Protein: 0g ‖ Carbohydrates: 25.5g ‖ Fat: 0g

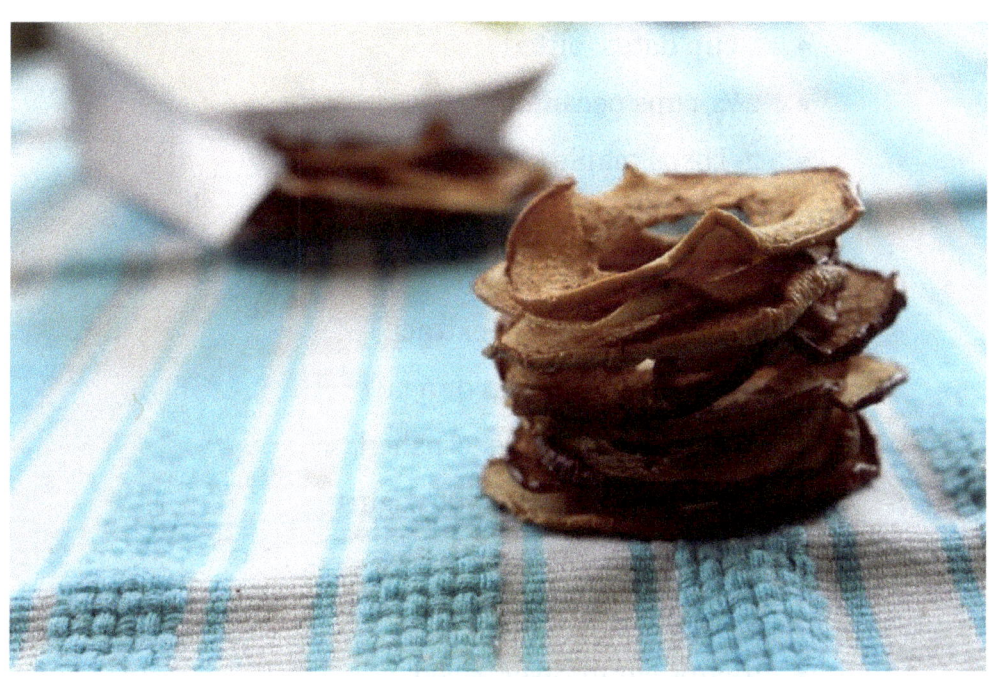

Citrus Cauliflower Cake

Time To Prepare: 5 hours and thirty minutes
Time to Cook: 0 minutes
Yield: Servings 10

Ingredients:
For the Crust:
- 1-cup dates, pitted
- 2½-cups pecan nuts
- 2-Tbsps maple syrup or agave

For the Filling:
- ½-tsp lemon extract
- ½-tsp pure vanilla extract
- ¾-cup maple syrup or agave
- 1½-cups pineapple, crushed
- 1½-cups plain coconut yogurt
- 1-pc lemon, zest, and juice
- 1-tsp pure vanilla extract
- 3-cups cauliflower, riced
- 3-pcs avocados, halved and pitted
- 3-Tbsps maple syrup or agave
- A pinch of cinnamon
- For the Topping:

Directions:
For the Crust:
1. Coat a baking tray using parchment paper. Set the outer ring of a 9-inch springform pan onto the baking tray.
2. Pulse the pecans in a food processor to a thoroughly ground texture. Put in the remaining crust ingredients, and pulse further until the mixture holds together.
3. Move and press the mixture to a uniform layer in the baking tray.

For the Filling:
1. Wipe the container of your food processor, and put in in the avocado, cauliflower, pineapple, syrup, and lemon zest and juice. Process the mixture to a smooth consistency.
2. Put in the cinnamon and the lemon and vanilla extracts. Pulse until meticulously blended. Pour the mixture over the crust. Put the tray in your freezer overnight, or for around five hours.
3. Take the cake out from your freezer, and allow it to sit at room temperature for about twenty minutes. Take away the outer ring.
4. For the Topping:

5. Mix in all the topping ingredients in a mixing container. Pour the mixture over the cake and spread uniformly.

Nutritional Info: ‖ Calories: 667 ‖ Fat: 22.2g ‖ Protein: 33.3g ‖ Sodium: 237mg ‖ Total Carbohydrates: 88.1g ‖ Fiber: 4.8g ‖ Net Carbohydrates: 83.3g

Citrus Strawberry Granita

Time To Prepare: fifteen minutes
Time to Cook: 0 minutes
Yield: Servings 4

Ingredients:

- ¼ cup of raw honey
- ¼ lemon
- 1 grapefruit (peeled, seeded, and sectioned)
- 12 ounces of fresh strawberries, hulled
- 2 oranges (peeled, seeded and sectioned)

Directions:

1. Put strawberries, grapefruit, oranges, and lemon in a juicer and extract juice according to the manufacturer's instructions.
2. Put 1½ cups of the veggie juice and honey to a pan and cook on moderate heat for five minutes while stirring constantly.
3. Remove it from heat and put in it to the rest of the juice.
4. Set aside for roughly thirty minutes.
5. Move the juice mixture into an 8x8-inch glass baking dish.

6. Freeze for 4 hours while scraping after every thirty minutes.

Nutritional Info: ‖ Calories: 145 ‖ Fat: 0.4g ‖ Carbohydrates: 37.5g ‖ Sugar: 32.4g ‖ Protein: 1.7g ‖ Sodium: 2mg

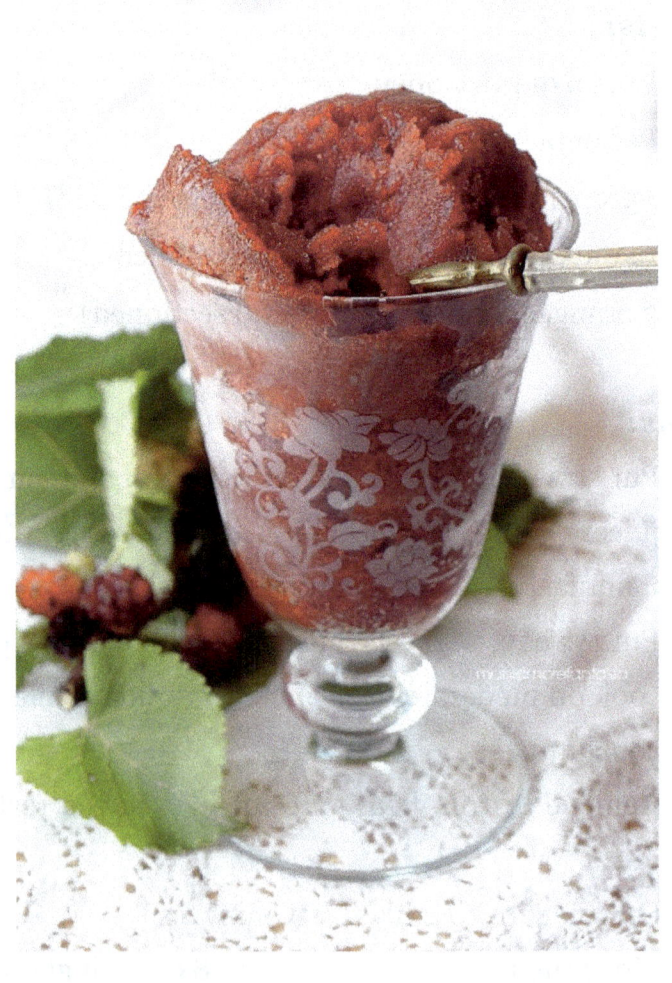

Coconut and Chocolate Cream

Time To Prepare: 2 hours
Time to Cook: 0 minutes
Yield: Servings 4

Ingredients:

- ½ teaspoon cinnamon powder
- 1 cup dark chocolate, chopped and melted
- 1 teaspoon vanilla extract
- 2 cups coconut milk
- 2 tablespoons ginger, grated
- 2 tablespoons honey

Directions:

Throw all the ingredients into a blender and blend. Split into bowls and store in the refrigerator for about two hours before you serve.

Nutritional Info: ‖ Calories: 200 ‖ Fat: 3 ‖ Fiber:5 ‖ Carbohydrates: 12 ‖ Protein: 7

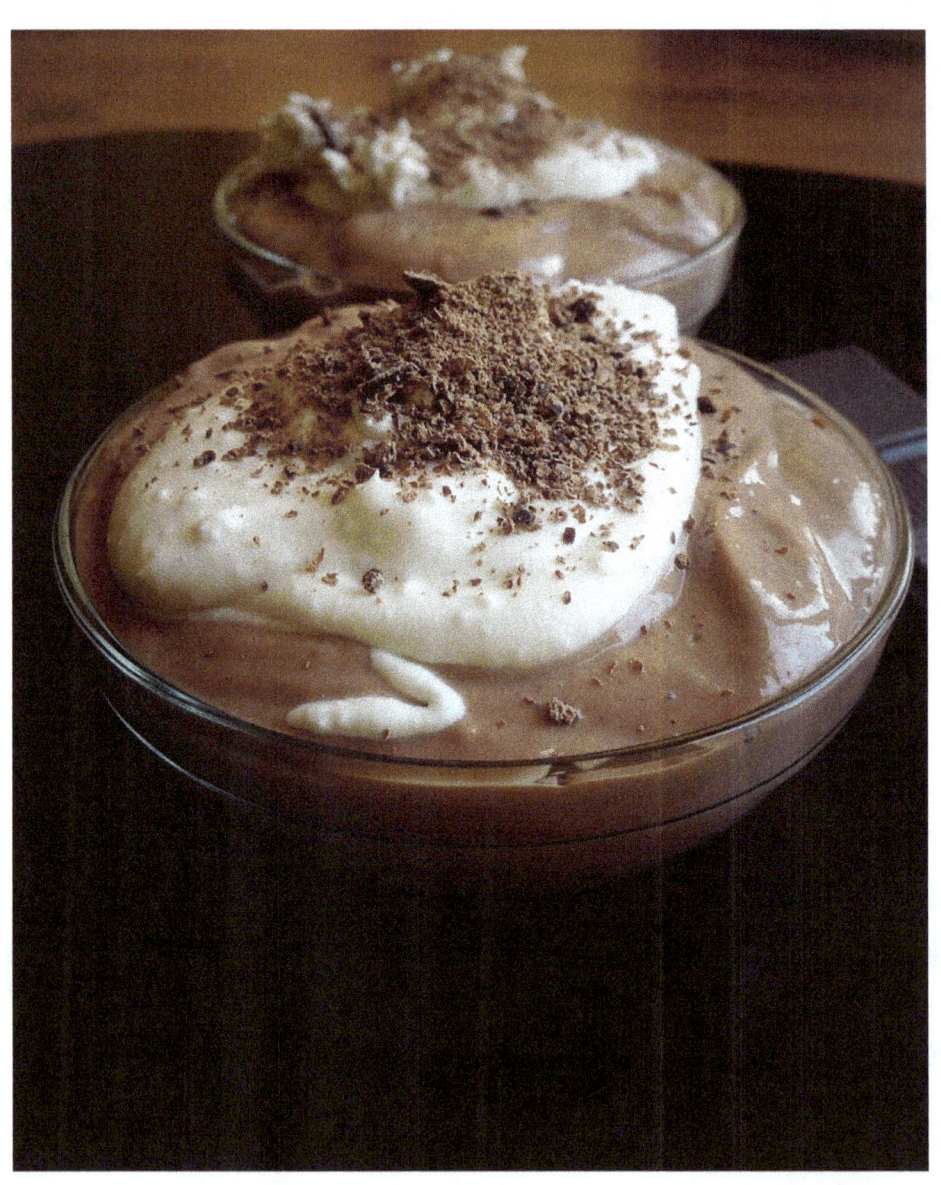

Coconut Butter Fudge

Time To Prepare: ten minutes
Time to Cook: 0 minutes
Yield: Servings 6

Ingredients:

- ¼ teaspoon of salt
- 1 cup of coconut butter
- 1 teaspoon of pure vanilla extract
- 2 tablespoons of raw honey

Directions:

1. Start by lining an 8 x 8 inch baking dish using parchment paper.
2. Melt the coconut butter, honey, and vanilla using low heat.
3. Place the mixture into the baking pan, and place in your fridge for about two hours before you serve.

Nutritional Info: ‖ Total Carbohydrates: 6g ‖ Fiber: 0g ‖ Net Carbohydrates: ‖ Protein: 0g ‖ Total Fat: 36g ‖ Calories: 334

Coconut Muffins

Time To Prepare: 5 Minutes
Time to Cook: 25 Minutes
Yield: Servings 8

Ingredients:

- ¼ cup of cocoa powder
- ¼ teaspoon vanilla extract
- ½ cup ghee, melted
- 1 cup coconut, unsweetened and shredded
- 1 teaspoon baking powder
- 3 tablespoons swerve
- eggs, whisked

Directions:

1. In a container, mix the ghee with the swerve, coconut, and the other ingredients, stir thoroughly and split it into a lined muffin pan.
2. Bake at 370 degrees F for about twenty-five minutes, cool down before you serve.

Nutritional Info: ‖ Calories: 324 ‖ Fat: 31g ‖ Carbohydrates: 8.3g ‖ Protein: 4g ‖ Sugar: 11g

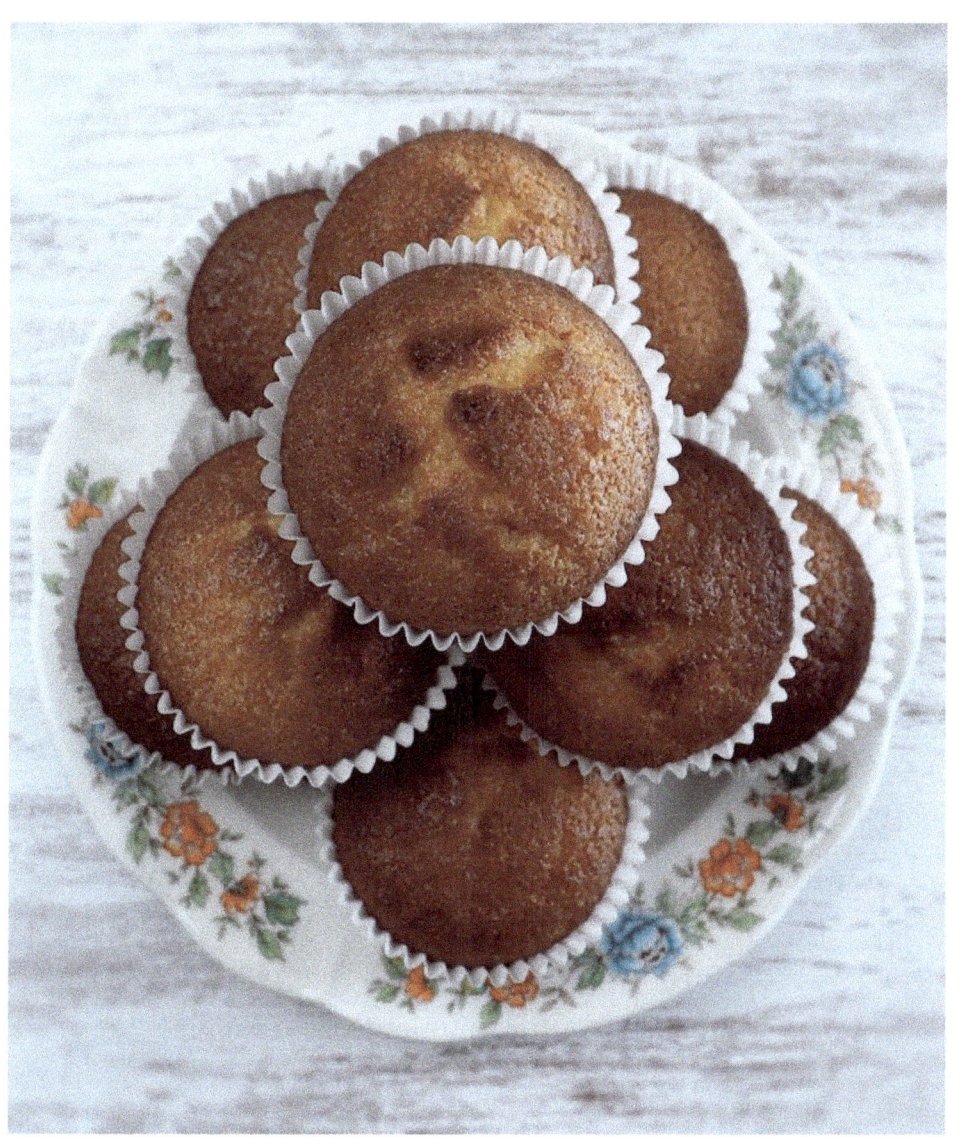

Coffee Cream

Time To Prepare: ten minutes
Time to Cook: fifteen minutes
Yield: Servings 4

Ingredients:

- ¼ cup brewed coffee
- 1 teaspoon vanilla extract
- 2 cups heavy cream
- 2 eggs
- 2 tablespoons ghee, melted
- 2 tablespoons swerve

Directions:

1. In a container, mix the coffee with the cream and the other ingredients, whisk well and split it into 4 ramekins and whisk well.
2. Introduce the ramekins in your oven at 350 degrees F and bake for fifteen minutes.
3. Serve warm.

Nutritional Info: Calories 300 ‖ Fat: 11g ‖ Carbohydrates: 3g ‖ Protein: 4g ‖ Sugar: 12g

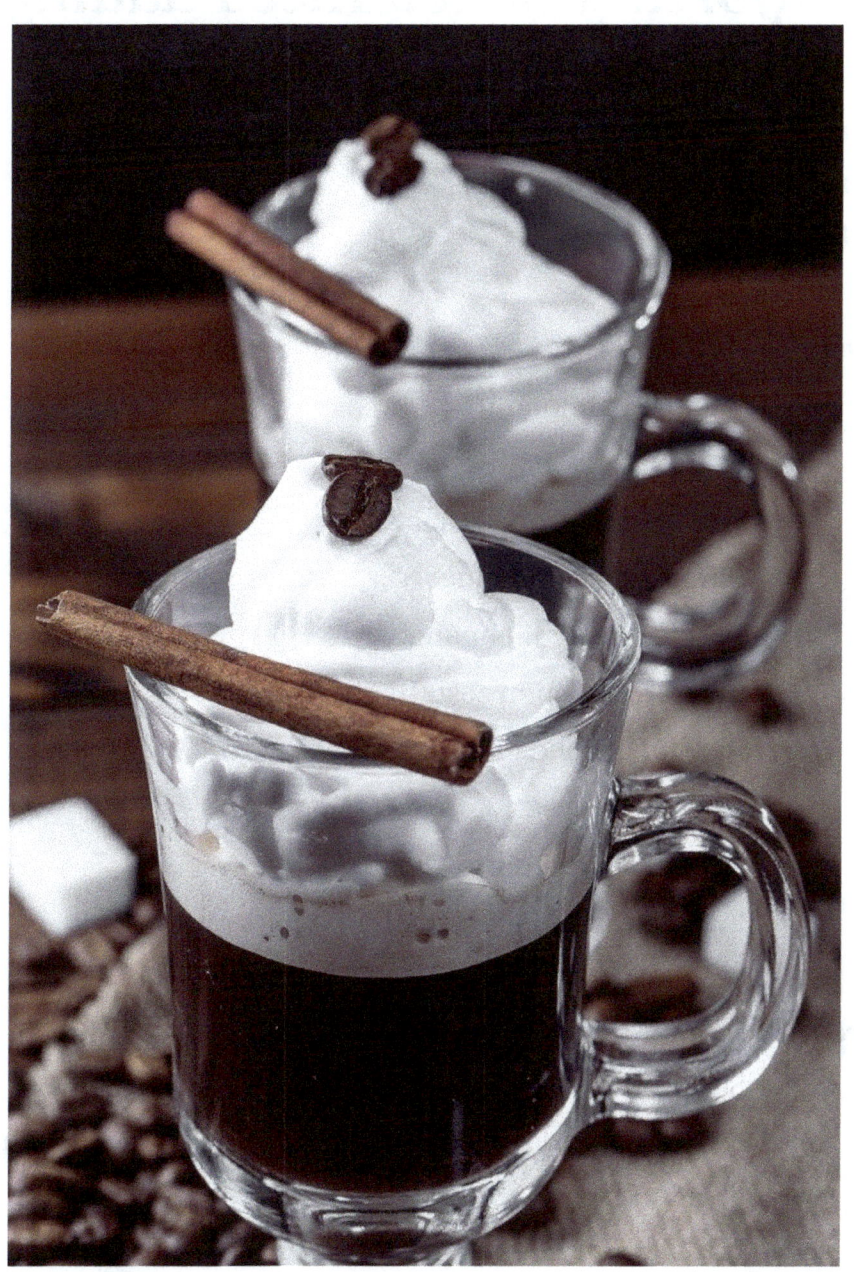

Comforting Baked Rice Pudding

Time To Prepare: ten minutes
Time to Cook: twenty minutes
Yield: Servings 8

Ingredients:

- ¼ cup of almond flakes
- ¼ cup of raw honey
- ½ tsp. of ground cardamom
- ½ tsp. of ground ginger
- 1 peeled and cut banana
- 1 tsp. fresh lemon zest, finely grated
- 1 tsp. of ground cinnamon
- 2 big organic eggs
- 2 cups of cooked brown rice
- 2 cups of unsweetened almond milk

Directions:

1. Set the oven to 390 F, then grease a baking dish.
2. Spread cooked rice at the bottom of the readied baking dish uniformly.
3. In a big container, put together the coconut milk, eggs, honey, lemon zest, spices, and beat until well blended.

4. Put the egg mixture over the rice uniformly.
5. Position banana slices over egg mixture uniformly and drizzle with almonds.
6. Bake for approximately twenty minutes.
7. Serve warm.

Nutritional Info: ‖ Calories: 264 ‖ Fat: 4.9g ‖ Carbohydrates: 50g ‖ Protein: 6.2g ‖ Fiber: 2.9g

Cookie Dough Bites

Time To Prepare: 10 Minutes
Time to Cook: 5 Minutes
Yield: Servings 2

Ingredients:

- ¼ cup Almond Flour
- ¼ cup Chocolate Chips, dairy-free & sugar-free
- ½ cup Almond Butter or any nut butter
- ½ tsp. Salt
- 1 ½ cups Chickpeas, cooked
- 1 tsp. Vanilla Extract
- 2 tbsp. Maple Syrup

Directions:

1. First, place all the ingredients excluding the chocolate chips in a high-speed blender for about three minutes or until you get a thick, smooth mixture.
2. After this, move the mixture to a moderate-sized container.
3. Next, fold in the chocolate chips into the batter.
4. Check for sweetness and put in more maple syrup if required.
5. Serve and enjoy.

Nutritional Info: ‖ Calories: 373 Kcal ‖ Protein: 12.6g ‖ Carbohydrates: 59.1g ‖ Fat:10g

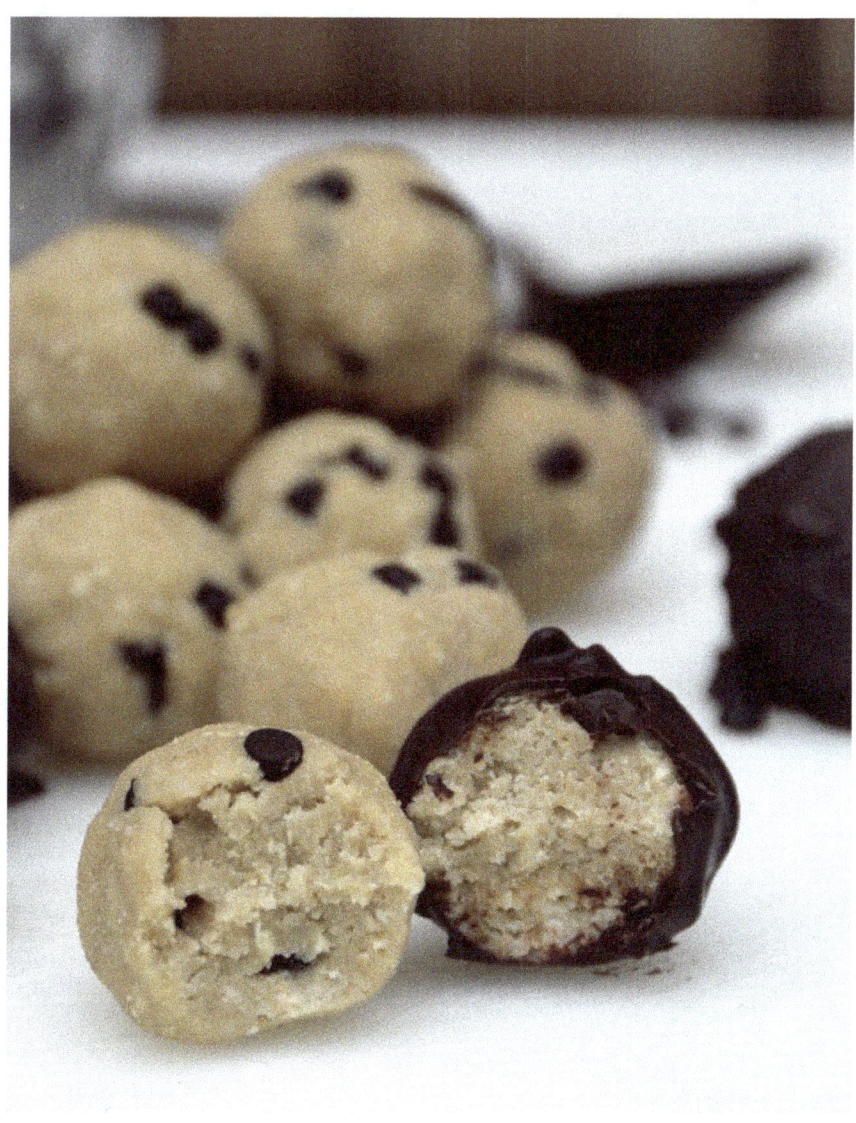

www.ingramcontent.com/pod-product-compliance
Lightning Source LLC
Chambersburg PA
CBHW070733030426
42336CB00013B/1954